GET
THROUGH

**Trauma
Examinations**

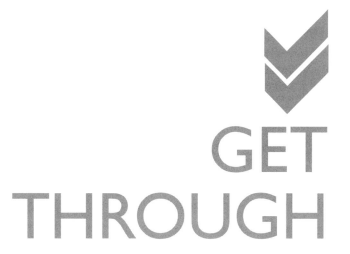

GET
THROUGH

Trauma
Examinations

James Wigley MBBS BSc MRCS AFHEA
University Hospital Southampton, Southampton, UK

Saran Shantikumar MRCS
BHF Research Fellow, Bristol Heart Institute, Bristol, UK

Andrew Paul Monk DPhil MRCS
Academic Clinical Lecturer in Orthopaedics
University of Oxford, Oxford, UK

Editorial Advisor

Stuart Blagg BSc FRCS FRCS (Tr & Orth)
Consultant Trauma and Orthopaedic Surgeon,
Stoke Mandeville Hospital, Buckinghamshire, UK

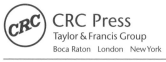 CRC Press
Taylor & Francis Group
Boca Raton   London   New York

CRC Press is an imprint of the
Taylor & Francis Group, an **informa** business

CRC Press
Taylor & Francis Group
6000 Broken Sound Parkway NW, Suite 300
Boca Raton, FL 33487-2742

Printed on acid-free paper
Version Date: 20140124

International Standard Book Number-13: 978-1-4441-7662-9 (Paperback)

This book contains information obtained from authentic and highly regarded sources. While all reasonable efforts have been made to publish reliable data and information, neither the author[s] nor the publisher can accept any legal responsibility or liability for any errors or omissions that may be made. The publishers wish to make clear that any views or opinions expressed in this book by individual editors, authors or contributors are personal to them and do not necessarily reflect the views/opinions of the publishers. The information or guidance contained in this book is intended for use by medical, scientific or health-care professionals and is provided strictly as a supplement to the medical or other professional's own judgement, their knowledge of the patient's medical history, relevant manufacturer's instructions and the appropriate best practice guidelines. Because of the rapid advances in medical science, any information or advice on dosages, procedures or diagnoses should be independently verified. The reader is strongly urged to consult the drug companies' printed instructions, and their websites, before administering any of the drugs recommended in this book. This book does not indicate whether a particular treatment is appropriate or suitable for a particular individual. Ultimately it is the sole responsibility of the medical professional to make his or her own professional judgements, so as to advise and treat patients appropriately. The authors and publishers have also attempted to trace the copyright holders of all material reproduced in this publication and apologize to copyright holders if permission to publish in this form has not been obtained. If any copyright material has not been acknowledged please write and let us know so we may rectify in any future reprint.

Library of Congress Cataloging-in-Publication Data

Wigley, James.
    Get through trauma examinations / James Wigley, Saran Shantikumar, Andrew Paul Monk.
        pages cm
    "A CRC title."
    Includes bibliographical references and index.
    ISBN 978-1-4441-7662-9 (hardcover : alk. paper)
      1. Traumatology--Examinations, questions, etc. 2. Wounds and injuries--Examinations, questions, etc.
  3. Orthopedics--Examinations, questions, etc. I. Shantikumar, Saran. II. Monk, Andrew Paul. III. Title.

    RD93.W545 2014
    617.10076--dc23   2013048179

Visit the Taylor & Francis Web site at
http://www.taylorandfrancis.com

and the CRC Press Web site at
http://www.crcpress.com

CONTENTS

PREFACE

Welcome to *Get Through: Trauma Examinations*. Ahead lie 150 SBA (single best answer) questions arranged as three practice papers. Each paper comprises a breadth of trauma topics but you will see that we have included more questions on particular topics, to emphasize where most exams centre their focus.

I hope this book fulfills its aim in being a useful, informative revision aid. If you have any feedback or suggestions, please let me know (james.wigley@gmail.com).

Finally, I would like to dedicate this book to my parents, and thank them for their endless support and inspiration over the years.

James Wigley

PAPER 1
QUESTIONS

Question 1

An oropharyngeal airway should be sized according to which one of the following descriptions?

A. The measurement between the canines and the angle of the jaw
B. The measurement between the labial commissure and the external auditory meatus
C. The approximate diameter of the patient's little finger
D. By a combination of the patient's sex and approximate size (big or small)
E. The measurement between the hyoid and the chin

Question 2

Before intubating a 28-year-old man, you aim to assess him for ease of intubation. Which of the following features would be suggestive of a difficult intubation?

A. Long neck
B. Distance of four fingers between the incisors with the mouth opened
C. Mallampati class I
D. An inability to rule out cervical spine fracture
E. Distance of two fingers between the thyroid notch and floor of the mouth

Question 3

A 41-year-old man has been attacked and has multiple stab wounds to the abdomen. He is pale and sweaty, and you see pools of blood collecting on the floor. His pulse is 140/min. His systolic blood pressure is 85 mmHg.
On arrival into the emergency department what is your first priority?

A. Insert large bore peripheral cannula to each antecubital fossa
B. Check his airway
C. Elevate his legs in order to increase venous return
D. Apply pressure to the laceration that you see is contributing to the blood loss
E. Quickly turn the patient over to see if there are further wounds

Question 4

A 32-year-old man is brought into the emergency department following a high-speed collision with a truck. He is complaining of severe left-sided chest pain. You note he is breathless, tachycardic and hypotensive. On examination there is reduced air entry on the left side and the trachea is deviated to the right. Which of the following is the most appropriate course of action?

A. Insert a chest drain into the fifth intercostal space left-hand side
B. Insert a wide bore cannula into the second intercostal space left-hand side
C. Request an urgent chest X-ray
D. Request an urgent ECG
E. Perform a pericardiocentesis

Question 5

A 21-year-old woman is admitted following a road traffic collision. She is dyspnoeic and has haemoptysis. On examination there is reduced air entry on the left with hyperresonance to percussion and evidence of subcutaneous emphysema. No penetrating wound is apparent.
Which of the following is the most likely underlying cause of her symptoms?

A. Aortic disruption
B. Diaphragmatic injury
C. Haemothorax
D. Tracheobronchial tree injury
E. Pulmonary contusion

Question 6

Which of the following ECG changes are commonly found following a myocardial contusion?

A. Atrial fibrillation
B. Multiple ventricular ectopics
C. Right bundle branch block
D. Sinus tachycardia
E. All of the above

Question 7

A 67-year-old man is being evaluated for brain death. The following features are noted: the gag reflex is absent, the GCS is 3, the core temperature is 34°C, the pupils are not reactive and there is no spontaneous ventilatory effort.
Which of the documented features preclude a diagnosis of brain death being given?

A. The gag reflex is absent
B. The GCS is 3
C. The core temperature is 34°C
D. The pupils are not reactive
E. There is no spontaneous respiratory effort

Question 8

Which of the following statements is FALSE with regard to cerebral blood flow?

A. Cerebral perfusion pressure is equal to mean arterial blood pressure minus intracranial pressure
B. Mean arterial blood pressure is equal to diastolic blood pressure plus 1/3 (systolic blood pressure–diastolic blood pressure)
C. A reduction in intracerebral pressure can be caused by raising the partial pressure of carbon dioxide
D. A normal intracranial pressure is equal to approximately 10–15 mmHg
E. Secondary brain injury is preventable

Question 9

A heavy goods vehicle ploughs into the rear of a car. Inside the car is a 72-year-old female who, following the crash, develops these clinical signs: power in the upper limbs 2/5, power in the lower limbs 4/5.
What is the most likely diagnosis?

A. Central cord syndrome
B. Anterior cord syndrome
C. Brown-Séquard syndrome
D. Complete transection of the cervical spinal cord
E. More information is required to make a diagnosis

Question 10

The immediate management of displaced fractures requires which of the following?

A. Realignment without splintage
B. Realignment and splintage
C. Immobilization in the most comfortable position
D. Splinting in the position they are found
E. Applying compression dressings

Question 11

A pregnant woman of 35 weeks has been assaulted. She has been stabbed in the left anterolateral abdominal wall. The appropriate steps have been made with regard to managing her airway and breathing. She remains hypotensive.
What should be the next step in her management?

A. Log roll the patient to the left and insert a wedge on the right-hand side so she remains at a tilt of 15 degrees in the supine position
B. Obtain a CTG to ensure the health of the foetus
C. Elevate the legs
D. Transfer the patient to the theatre immediately
E. Consider the use of vasopressors

Question 12

The hangman's fracture involves which of the following vertebral areas?

A. Occipito-cervical junction
B. C1
C. C2
D. C3
E. Cervico-thoracic junction

Question 13

A 70-year-old man has been involved in a cyclist versus car collision. He has sustained a fracture to his second lumbar vertebrae. His haemoglobin on admission was measured at 11.9 g/dl. Two hours later you are called to review him by the nursing staff, as he looks pale and sweaty. Repeat bloods reveal a haemoglobin of 6.4 g/dl. Of note, a FAST scan was performed on admission and reported as normal.
Of the following options, what is the next most appropriate step in the management of this patient?

A. Reassure the nurses that the full blood count is a consequence of dilution from fluid resuscitation
B. Repeat the blood test again as it is likely to be an erroneous result
C. Arrange prompt angiography
D. Fluid challenge with 1 litre of 5% dextrose
E. Arrange a CT of abdomen and pelvis

Question 14

Which is the most accurate way to calculate the body surface area of burns in children?

A. Lund & Browder charts
B. Using the patient's palm (equates to 1% body surface area)
C. Wallace's 'rule of nines'
D. Measure the area with a tape measure
E. The Parkland formula

Question 15

A patient who was recently admitted to your emergency department following a road traffic collision requires transfer to a tertiary centre of care. A primary survey has been completed and some problems are noted that require intervention. Which of the following necessary interventions should be addressed prior to transfer?

A. Remove large foreign bodies from skin wounds
B. Obtain X-rays of open ankle fracture
C. Insert an indwelling catheter
D. Obtain haemodynamic stability
E. Clear the C-spine

Question 16

The American Burn Association has identified several types of thermal injury that typically require transfer to a burn centre.
Which of the following is NOT such a criterion?

A. >10% burns in any age group
B. Any burn in patients under 10 years
C. Facial burns
D. Full-thickness burns >5%
E. Inhalation injuries

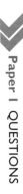

Question 17

A motorcyclist has been involved in a collision with a car at high speed. While en route to the hospital he has received 1 litre of crystalloid. His systolic blood pressure is 80 mmHg and increases to 85 mmHg with a further litre of normal saline in the emergency department. The patient is awake and describes to you how the accident happened.

Before the patient is log rolled, which of the following should be done next?

A. Consider blood products and rapidly assess the patient for a source of bleeding
B. Insert a urethral catheter so an hourly urine output can be determined
C. Obtain further intravenous access so two bags of crystalloid can be infused rapidly and simultaneously
D. Continue to replenish fluids with crystalloids at a reduced speed
E. 'Group and save' the patient

Question 18

A 24-year-old man presents after a fight and is suspected of having bilateral mandible fractures. He begins to develop respiratory distress.
What position for ongoing resuscitation should be considered in this patient?

A. Left lateral position
B. Right lateral position
C. Supine
D. Sitting upright
E. Trendelenburg

Question 19

A 59-year-old woman is involved in a motor collision. On arrival at the hospital she is short of breath and complains of left-sided chest pain. On examination there is an area of paradoxical movement of the chest wall.
Which of the following would be the most appropriate management option given the likely diagnosis?

A. Oxygen, analgesia and respiratory support
B. Chest drain insertion
C. Emergency thoracotomy
D. Immediate intubation
E. Pericardiocentesis

Question 20

Which of the following statements is FALSE?

A. A fracture of the fifth rib can give rise to penetrating intra-abdominal injury
B. The aponeurotic sheaths of the anterior abdominal wall are relative weak points compared with the musculature that surrounds the lateral and posterior abdomen
C. Diagnostic peritoneal lavage is effective at detecting blood loss within the retroperitoneum
D. Patients can lose a significant amount of blood within the abdominal cavity despite displaying no features of peritonism
E. The diaphragm marks the superior border of the abdominal cavity

Question 21

A 45-year-old man is brought to the emergency room after a fall from a balcony. On arrival he makes no sound, does not open his eyes to pain and makes no motor response to stimuli.
What is his Glasgow Coma Score?

A. 0
B. 1
C. 3
D. 5
E. 7

Question 22

A 42-year-old man is brought to the emergency department following a road traffic collision. On arrival, you note that he is immobilized in a hard collar, has facial fractures and is in acute respiratory distress. An attempt at orotracheal tube insertion is unsuccessful.
Which of the following would be the next step in his airway management?

A. Re-attempt orotracheal intubation after 5 minutes
B. Attempt nasotracheal intubation
C. Perform a cricothyroidotomy
D. Attempt laryngeal mask airway insertion
E. Perform a tracheostomy

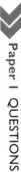

Question 23

Which of the following is considered a normal intracranial pressure in the resting state?

A. 1 mmHg
B. 5 mmHg
C. 9 mmHg
D. 17 mmHg
E. 22 mmHg

Question 24

In a patient with a C-spine fracture identified following a primary survey, what is the likelihood of a second, non-contiguous fracture?

A. 5%
B. 10%
C. 25%
D. 50%
E. 75%

Question 25

A 23-year-old man has been smashed over the head with a beer bottle. He opens his eyes as fragments of glass are removed from his scalp. He is groaning as he tries to stop your rubbing his sternum by raising his right arm and moving it towards you.
What is his Glasgow Coma Score?

A. 7
B. 8
C. 9
D. 10
E. 11

Question 26

Which of the following is the most common cause of a tension pneumothorax?

A. Markedly displaced thoracic spine fractures
B. Penetrating chest trauma
C. Positive pressure ventilation in patients with visceral pleural injury
D. Spontaneous rupture of an emphysematous bulla
E. Subclavian vein catheterization

Question 27

You are prescribing crystalloid intravenous fluid resuscitation for a 40-year-old man who has sustained a 15% second-degree burn to his chest. You decide to give 2 ml/kg. The patient weighs 80 kg.
What rate of infusion should be prescribed?

A. 50 ml/hr
B. 100 ml/hr
C. 150 ml/hr
D. 200 ml/hr
E. 250 ml/hr

Question 28

An inner city shopkeeper is shot in the abdomen.
Which of the following statements is FALSE?

A. Fifty percent of gunshot wounds to the abdomen involve the small bowel
B. Exit wounds from a gunshot will be located in a line made from the pistol and the entry wound
C. Handguns represent a medium energy penetrating injury
D. The amount of damage caused by a bullet is dependent upon the transfer of energy to the tissue, the duration of energy transfer and the amount of tissue involved
E. The damage caused by a shotgun diminishes considerably if fired from a distance of 3 metres or more

Question 29

Which of the following statements about cerebral blood flow is FALSE?

A. Brain injury may result in an acute drop in cerebral blood flow
B. Cerebral blood flow is reduced by hypotension, hypoxia and hypocapnia
C. During childhood, cerebral blood flow can reach 90 ml/minute/100 g brain tissue
D. The normal cerebral blood flow in healthy adults is 20 ml/minute/100 g brain tissue
E. The cerebral perfusion pressure is calculated by the mean arterial pressure minus the intracranial pressure

Question 30

A 21-year-old man is brought to the emergency department after being stabbed in the chest. He is visibly tachypnoeic and on examination has a large sucking wound to the left side of the chest.
Which of the following is not an appropriate management option?

A. Analgesia
B. Chest drain insertion
C. Oxygen supplementation
D. Sterile occlusive dressing over the wound
E. Surgical airway

Question 31

What is the likelihood of a patient with a traumatic brain injury having an associated spinal injury?

A. 1%
B. 2%
C. 5%
D. 25%
E. 55%

Question 32

The highest achievable eye opening score on the Glasgow Coma Scale is:

A. 1
B. 2
C. 3
D. 4
E. 5

Question 33

The most common region for spinal injuries to occur is:

A. Cervical
B. Thoracic
C. Thoracolumbar junction
D. Lumbar
E. Lumbar–sacral junction

Question 34

An assessment of the musculoskeletal system forms part of which of the following?

A. Primary survey
B. Secondary survey
C. Choice of adjunct
D. History
E. All of the above

Question 35

Which of the following is not consistent with the mechanism of injury?

A. Air bag: corneal abrasion and cardiac rupture
B. Shoulder harness: pulmonary contusion and intimal tear or thrombosis of subclavian artery
C. Lap seatbelt: Chance fracture of lumbar spine
D. Rear end shunt: hyperextension of the cervical spine with multiple laminar, pedicle and spinous process fractures
E. Pedestrian versus cyclist: deceleration injury

Question 36

Helpful information for the receiving institution of a patient transfer includes which of the following?

A. Patient demographic details
B. AMPLE history
C. Status and previous management
D. Diagnostic investigations
E. All of the above

Question 37

In patients with spinal immobilization in place, how often should a log roll be performed to minimize the risk of pressure sores?

A. Every 30 minutes
B. Every 45 minutes
C. Every 1 hour
D. Every 2 hours
E. Every 4 hours

Question 38

A typical closed long bone fracture results in what approximate volume of blood loss?

A. 1 litre
B. 2 litres
C. 3 litres
D. 4 litres
E. Greater than 5 litres

Question 39

An 18-year-old man is involved in a fire at work. He has full-thickness burns over both his arms and partial thickness burns over the whole of the front torso. Estimate the percentage burn he has sustained.

A. 18%
B. 27%
C. 30%
D. 36%
E. 45%

Question 40

Regarding the unique characteristics of paediatric patients, which of the following statements is FALSE?

A. Hypothermia tends to develop more quickly
B. Injuries in a child can result in personality and emotional disturbances in uninjured siblings
C. Injuries through growth plates may result in subsequent growth abnormalities
D. Internal organ damage is often seen without overlying bony fracture
E. Around 10% of children who sustain severe multisystem trauma have residual personality changes at 1 year

Question 41

Pertinent questions from the history regarding musculoskeletal trauma include which of the following?

A. Involvement of police
B. Time of day
C. Post-crash location of the patient
D. Height of patient
E. Time patient last ate or drank

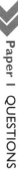

Question 42

A 42-year-old woman is brought in after a road traffic collision. You notice that she is hypoxic and struggling to ventilate. Palpation of the neck is abnormal.
Which of the following most specifically suggests a laryngeal fracture?

A. Subcutaneous emphysema
B. Distended neck veins
C. Inability to palpate the fracture
D. Tachycardia
E. No change in the quality of the voice

Question 43

A 42-year-old woman has accidentally spilled hot oil from a frying pan over her left hand. On examination in the emergency room, you notice a dry, dark area of skin over the dorsum of the hand, which appears leathery. There is a demonstrable absence of pain from this area.
How is the depth of the burn best described?

A. First degree
B. Superficial
C. Second degree
D. Partial thickness
E. Full thickness

Question 44

A secondary survey is required in which of the following scenarios?

A. Isolated head injuries
B. Isolated fracture (non-long bone)
C. Thoracic trauma
D. Abdominal trauma
E. All of the above

Question 45

During the assessment of muscle strength, what does a score of 4 represent?

A. Total paralysis
B. Full range of motion with gravity eliminated
C. Full range of motion against gravity
D. Full range of motion but less than normal strength
E. Non-testable

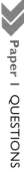

Question 46

A 29-year-old man is admitted to the emergency department after a fall from his bike, which resulted in a head injury. On examination his eyes open spontaneously, he is able to obey commands and his verbal response is orientated.
How would his brain injury be classified?

A. Very minor
B. Minor
C. Moderate
D. Severe
E. Life-threatening

Question 47

You come across an injured motorcyclist following a road traffic collision. He is wearing a helmet. You are keen to remove this in order to perform an airway maintenance manoeuvre.
How should the helmet be removed?

A. One person: gently slide the helmet from the head in the supine position
B. One person: rotate the neck to one side before sliding the helmet off
C. Two people: one person provides in-line stabilization of the head and neck, the other removes the helmet in the supine position
D. Two people: one person provides in-line stabilization of the head and neck, the other instructs the patient on how to remove the helmet himself
E. Three people: one person provides in-line stabilization of the head and neck, one holds the patient's feet, one removes the helmet in the supine position

Question 48

Severe injury following major pelvic disruption can be due to which of the following?

A. Arterial damage
B. Venous damage
C. Fracture
D. Pelvic organ damage
E. All of the above

Question 49

Regarding carbon monoxide inhalation, which of the following statements is TRUE?

A. A cherry-red skin discolouration is common
B. Inhalation of even small quantities usually results in headaches
C. Intubation is mandatory
D. It cannot result in coma
E. Treatment with 100% oxygen increases the rate of dissociation of carboxyhaemoglobin

Question 50

Which of the following nerve palsies is not associated with the preceding injuries?

A. Fibular neck fracture: superficial peroneal nerve
B. Anterior shoulder dislocation: ulnar nerve
C. Acetabular fracture: superior and inferior gluteal nerve
D. Supracondylar fractures in children: median and anterior interosseous nerve
E. Knee dislocation: posterior tibial nerve

2

Answer 1: B. The measurement of the labial commissure to the external auditory meatus

Oropharyngeal (or Guedel) tubes are a type of airway adjunct. The correct size is selected by measuring the airway against the patient's head, either between the corner of the mouth (labial commissure) and the external auditory meatus, or from the angle of the jaw to the incisors. A nasopharyngeal tube is sized by approximating the diameter of the patient's little finger. Laryngeal mask airways (LMAs) are sized according to the approximate patient size and sex, as follows:

- LMA size 3: small women
- LMA size 4: large women or small man
- LMA size 5: large man

The measurement between the hyoid and the chin is part of the 3-3-2 rule in the assessment of a difficult intubation (see answer 2).

Arthur Ernest Guedel, American anaesthetist (1883–1956)

Answer 2: D. An inability to rule out cervical spine fracture

The LEMON assessment can be used to predict difficult intubation, as follows. L = look externally for characteristics that are known to cause difficult intubation or ventilation, such as a short, muscular neck, a receding chin or an overbite. E = evaluate the 3-3-2 rule as follows: the distance between the incisors should be 3 finger breadths; the distance between the hyoid bone and chin should be at least 3 finger breadths; and the distance between the thyroid notch and floor of the mouth should be at least 2 finger breadths. M = Mallampati score, as follows: class 1 – soft palate, uvula, fauces and pillars visible; class 2 – soft palate, uvula, fauces (but not pillars) visible; class 3 – soft palate and base of uvula visible; class 4 – hard palate only visible. O = obstruction: any cause that can cause airway obstruction, and thus make laryngoscopy and ventilation difficult (e.g. trauma, peritonsillar abscess). N = neck mobility: reduced neck mobility makes intubation difficult and immobilized patients in a hard collar (such as trauma patients in

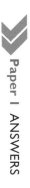

whom a cervical spine fracture has not yet been ruled out) will clearly have no neck movement.

The Mallampati score, published in 1985 by the *Canadian Anaesthetists' Society Journal*, was named after Seshagiri Mallampati, an American anaesthetist.

Answer 3: B. Check his airway

This patient's presentation carries the risk of airway or breathing problems. Always follow a logical progression of ABCDE. This reduces the chance of important injuries being missed and allows all involved to manage the most imminent threat to life first. All the answers here with the exception of option B address circulation and exposure.

Answer 4: B. Insert a wide bore cannula into the second intercostal space left-hand side

This patient has a tension pneumothorax. Air entering the pleural cavity during inspiration cannot escape during expiration due to the pleura acting as a one-way valve. Tension pneumothorax is an emergency, as the build-up of air compresses the lung, preventing expansion. This puts pressure on the mediastinum, reducing cardiac output, which can be potentially fatal if not relieved. Symptoms include breathlessness and chest pain, and on examination there is tachypnoea, hypotension, reduced expansion and air entry on the affected side of the chest, hyperresonance to percussion on the affected side and deviation of the trachea and apex beat to the opposite side. If not decompressed urgently, cardiorespiratory collapse and death can ensue within minutes. Decompression is by insertion of a large bore cannula into the second intercostal space in the mid-clavicular line of the affected side (needle thoracocentesis). A gush of air will be heard as the pressure is released. A formal chest drain can then be inserted (fifth intercostal space of the mid-axillary line). Do not waste time obtaining a chest X-ray or ECG if the diagnosis is suspected. Treatment should be based on clinical findings.

Answer 5: D. Tracheobronchial tree injury

This patient has an injury to the tracheobronchial tree. None of the other given options would result in the clinical findings described. Injuries to the tracheobronchial tree are unusual and associated with a high early mortality. Clinical features include haemoptysis and subcutaneous emphysema, as well as those associated with a tension pneumothorax. After chest drain insertion, a large persistent air leak is common and more than one tube may be required to overcome a large leak. Temporary intubation of the contralateral main bronchus may be possible, but operative intervention is a priority.

Answer 6: E. All of the above

Blunt injury to the chest can result in a myocardial contusion. Dysrhythmias are typical. The most common ECG findings are multiple ventricular ectopics, sinus tachycardia, atrial fibrillation, ST-segment changes and bundle branch block (usually on the right). Affected patients should be closely monitored for life-threatening dysrhythmias for 24 hours. After this interval, the risk of dysrhythmias decreases substantially.

Answer 7: C. The core temperature is 34°C

The diagnosis of brain death requires the following criteria to be satisfied: GCS of 3, pupils are non-reactive, there should be no spontaneous ventilatory effort, and the brainstem reflexes must be absent (e.g. oculocephalic, corneal, doll's eyes and gag reflexes). Ancillary studies that may be used to confirm brain death include: EEG (no activity at high gain), cerebral blood flow (none), intracranial pressure (should exceed mean arterial pressure for an hour) and cerebral angiography. Hypothermia and barbiturate intoxication can mimic brain death and hence must be excluded. As this patient's temperature is 34°C, he should be warmed and a diagnosis of brain death provided only if the criteria are fulfilled at normothermia.

Answer 8: C. A reduction in intracerebral pressure can be caused by raising the partial pressure of carbon dioxide

This question deals with the Monroe-Kelly doctrine, which describes the brain located inside a solid box (the skull). It explains how the pressure inside this box (intracerebral pressure) will rise once the compensatory mechanisms have been overcome. Secondary brain injury can be prevented by ensuring adequate oxygenation of the brain, and that carbon dioxide levels do not rise above normal limits.

A raised $PaCO_2$ causes intracranial vasodilatation and a further increase in intracranial pressure.

Alexander Monroe, Scottish surgeon (1733–1817)
George Kelly, Scottish anatomist (18th century)

Answer 9: A. Central cord syndrome

This vignette describes a classic central cord syndrome resulting from a rear end shunt and hyperflexion injury. The pathogenesis describes a vascular insufficiency from the anterior spinal artery. The artery supplies the central part of the cord. The arrangement of the motor fibres of the cervical cord causes the upper limbs to be most severely affected.

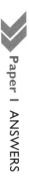

Brown-Séquard syndrome describes the features of unilateral transection (hemisection) of the spinal cord. Affected patients suffer ipsilateral loss of motor function with impaired joint position and vibration sense (dorsal column dysfunction). There is also a contralateral sensory loss for pain and temperature. Brown-Séquard syndrome has the best prognosis of all spinal cord lesions.

Charles-Édouard Brown-Séquard, British neurologist (1817–1894)

Answer 10: B. Realignment and splintage

The initial management of displaced fractures should be performed following manipulation into the anatomical position. Realignment is achieved using in-line traction. The main role of the splint is to prevent any further damage to the soft tissue structures including nerves, arteries and veins. If closed reduction of a dislocated joint is unsuccessful it is perfectly reasonable to only splint the deformity.

Answer 11: A. Log roll the patient to the left and insert a wedge on the right-hand side so she remains at a tilt of 15 degrees in the supine position

This woman is heavily pregnant. A large uterus can compress the inferior vena cava and result in impaired venous return. As Starling's law predicts, reduced pre-load results in a reduction in contractility, cardiac output and a subsequent drop in blood pressure. The best way to ensure the health of the foetus is to optimize the health of the mother. Vasopressors have a detrimental effect on the foetus by reducing uterine blood flow.

Answer 12: C. C2

A hangman's fracture involves the posterior elements of C2 at the pars interarticularis.

Answer 13: C. Arrange prompt angiography

Elderly patients admitted with trauma should be closely monitored. Lack of physiological reserve and co-morbidities makes for a more guarded prognosis than younger individuals.

The low haemoglobin result should be viewed with respect to the clinical picture. Sympathetic overdrive caused by inadequate resuscitation will lead to peripheral vasoconstriction of the skin and perspiration.

Retroperitoneal bleeding is a common unrecognized source of bleeding. A FAST scan will not detect retroperitoneal haemorrhage. In this circumstance the patient should undergo immediate angiography with attempted transcatheter embolization.

If a fall in haemoglobin is caused by dilution, urea and packed cell volume will also be decreased.

Answer 14: A. Lund & Browder charts

Lund & Browder charts are widely used in clinical practice and offer an accurate way of assessing the percentage body surface area of burns. Areas of skin with erythema and no blistering should not be included in the calculation. Wallace's 'rule of nines' is easier to remember and use, but less accurate. Knowing that the surface area of the patient's palm equates to 1% of the total body surface area can also be useful.

Once the percentage body surface area of burn is known, an accurate calculation can be made of the volume of fluid that should be used for resuscitation. The Parkland formula can be used for this.

Answer 15: D. Obtain haemodynamic stability

The principle of immediate trauma management is to perform the primary survey and, where required, address issues prior to immediate transfer. Remember, 'life before limb'.

Answers A, B, C and E would be performed either during the secondary survey or later. During the primary survey, the C-spine would be protected using collar and blocks, but not necessarily definitively cleared.

Answer 16: B. Any burn in patients under 10 years

Transferring all patients under the age of 10 with minor burns would be an inappropriate use of resources.

The American Burn Association gives the following list of types of burn injury that require transfer to a burn centre:
1. Partial-thickness and full-thickness burns on greater than 10% of the body surface area in any patient
2. Partial-thickness and full-thickness burns involving the face, eyes, ears, hands, feet, genitalia, and perineum, as well as those that involve skin overlying major joints
3. Full-thickness burns of any size in any age group
4. Significant electrical burns, including lightning injury (significant volumes of tissue beneath the surface can be injured and result in acute renal failure and other complications)
5. Significant chemical burns
6. Inhalation injury
7. Burn injury in patients with pre-existing illness that could complicate treatment, prolong recovery, or affect mortality

8. Any patient with a burn injury who has concomitant trauma poses an increased risk of morbidity or mortality, and may be treated initially in a trauma centre until stable before being transferred to a burn centre
9. Children with burn injuries who are seen in hospitals without qualified personnel or equipment to manage their care should be transferred to a burn centre with these capabilities
10. Burn injury in patients will require specialized social and emotional or long-term rehabilitative support, including cases involving suspected child maltreatment and neglect

Answer 17: A. Consider blood products and rapidly assess the patient for a source of bleeding

The patient is almost certainly haemorrhaging from somewhere but is perfusing his vital organs adequately at this stage as evidenced by his appropriate narrative of what happened. Be aware though that young and fit patients may perfuse their brain with a loss of up to 50% of their circulating volume, and then crash. This question aims to address the valid risk of over-transfusing with crystalloid in hypovolaemic shock.

Answer 18: D. Sitting upright

Bilateral mandibular fractures can cause a loss of normal airway support. For this reason, airway obstruction can result if the patient is in a supine position. Remember that the patient who refuses to lie flat may be having difficulty maintaining their airway, and those with bilateral mandible fractures would be best nursed sitting upright. Obviously, this can only be done after ruling out cervical spine injury, and a definitive airway may be necessary.

The Trendelenburg position describes the patient lying supine with the feet elevated above the head. It would therefore exacerbate the problem here. The left lateral position is useful in pregnant patients, as this relieves the pressure of the gravid uterus from the inferior vena cava, thus improving venous return. There is no specific advantage of the right (as opposed to left) lateral decubitus position in the trauma setting.

Answer 19: A. Oxygen, analgesia and respiratory support

The examination findings suggest a flail chest. A flail chest is a life-threatening injury caused by high-impact trauma resulting in two or more consecutive ribs being broken in two or more places. That segment of the chest wall then moves independently, moving in on inspiration and out on expiration – so-called paradoxical motion. Flail chests may be associated with an underlying pulmonary contusion and there is a risk of pneumothorax from rupture of the pleura by bone ends. This injury is associated with a high mortality. The most important part of management is the administration of oxygen but, by improving patient comfort by providing adequate analgesia (such as intercostal nerve blocks), respiratory effort can also be improved. Depending on the degree of hypoxia, positive pressure ventilation may be required and its use has largely superseded rib fracture fixation. The mortality associated with a flail chest is largely dependent on the degree of the underlying pulmonary contusion.

Answer 20: C. Diagnostic peritoneal lavage is effective at detecting blood loss within the retroperitoneum

The identification of retroperitoneal bleeding can be clinically difficult, and DPL (diagnostic peritoneal lavage) would be inappropriate if such a suspicion was raised. If an injury to a retroperitoneal organ is suspected, a FAST scan (Focused Assessment with Sonography for Trauma) or CT imaging would be indicated. Retroperitoneal organs include the pancreas, duodenum, ureters, kidneys and posterior aspects of ascending and descending colons.

Answer 21: C. 3

Based on the Glasgow Coma Scale (below), this patient's score is E1 V1 M1. The Glasgow Coma Scale (GCS) is a subjective scale used for the initial and continuing assessment of levels of consciousness in patients presenting following brain injury. The components are as follows:

Eye opening (E)
   4   Eyes open spontaneously
   3   Eyes open to speech
   2   Eyes open to pain
   1   No eye opening

Best motor response (M)
   6   Obeys commands
   5   Localizes to pain
   4   Withdraws from pain (normal flexion)
   3   Abnormal flexion in response to pain (decorticate response)
   2   Abnormal extension in response to pain (decerebrate response)
   1   No motor response

Verbal response (V)
   5   Coherent speech
   4   Confused/disorientated speech
   3   Inappropriate words without conversational exchange
   2   Incomprehensible sounds
   1   No verbal response

   The maximum score is thus 15 (E4 M6 V5), and the minimum is 3 (E1 M1 V1). Hence a score of 0 or 1 is impossible.

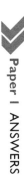

Answer 22: D. Attempt laryngeal mask airway insertion

The following airway decision scheme is for use in immobilized patients (i.e. suspected C-spine fracture) with apnoea or acute respiratory distress. If an attempt at orotracheal intubation is unsuccessful, it is best to proceed swiftly rather than wait and re-attempt it later. Given the patient's facial injuries, a nasotracheal tube should not be inserted. In this case a laryngeal mask airway (or other extraglottic device) should be inserted as a temporary bridge to a definitive airway. If this fails, a cricothyroidotomy should be performed.

Answer 23: C. 9 mmHg

The normal intracranial pressure (ICP) in the resting state is approximately 10 mmHg (7 to 15 mmHg). Many pathological processes that affect the brain may result in a raised ICP. A raised ICP in turn may reduce cerebral perfusion and cause or exacerbate cerebral ischaemia. A sustained ICP over 20 mmHg is associated with poorer outcomes.

Answer 24: B. 10%

Approximately 10% of patients with C-spine fractures have a second non-contiguous vertebral column fracture.

Answer 25: C. 9

This man is able to localize pain, open his eyes to noxious stimuli and is making incomprehensible sounds. This gives him a Glasgow Coma Score of 9 (Eyes 2, Verbal 2, Motor 5). Patients intoxicated with alcohol represent a challenge to the attending physician. NICE guidelines stipulate that if any of the following list be present, urgent CT imaging should be arranged. Note the fact that alcohol intoxication should have no bearing on the decision to image the brain.

The following is a list of indications for urgent neuroimaging:

- GCS <13 on initial assessment in the emergency department
- GCS <15 two hours after the injury on assessment in the emergency department
- Suspected open or depressed skull fracture
- Any sign of basal skull fracture, e.g.
  - Haemotympanum (blood behind the tympanic membrane)
  - 'Panda eyes' (bilateral periorbital ecchymosis caused by blood from ruptured venous sinuses tracking into the cranial sinuses, aka 'raccoon eyes')
  - Bilateral subconjunctival haemorrhage
  - Cerebrospinal fluid leakage from ears (CSF otorrhoea) or nose (CSF rhinorrhoea)
  - Battle's sign (perimastoid ecchymosis from extravasation of blood along the path of the posterior auricular artery)

- Post-traumatic seizure
- Focal neurological deficit
- >1 episode of vomiting
- Amnesia for events more than 30 minutes before the injury

William Henry Battle, English surgeon (1855–1936)

The Glasgow Coma Score was first published in 1974 by Graham Teasdale and Bryan Jennett, both professors of neurosurgery at the University of Glasgow. Note there is a modified version of the scale: a 14-point scale that omits 'abnormal flexion'. The modified scale is also in use, including at the founding unit in Glasgow.

Answer 26: C. Positive pressure ventilation in patients with visceral pleural injury

The most common cause of a tension pneumothorax is mechanical ventilation, specifically with positive pressure ventilation in patients with visceral pleural injury. In these cases it may be difficult to spot as the patient is typically sedated. It can also occur as a complication of a simple pneumothorax following penetrating or blunt chest injuries where the parenchymal lung injury fails to seal. Other causes include attempted subclavian/internal jugular venous catheter insertion, poor occlusive dressings in open chest wounds that create a flap-valve and markedly displaced thoracic spine fractures.

Answer 27: C. 150 ml/hr

In accordance with ATLS guidelines, patients with significant burns require 2 to 4 ml/kg of intravenous fluid resuscitation per percentage of second-/third-degree burn in the first 24 hours. Half of this is given in the first 8 hours, and the second half is given over the subsequent 16 hours. In this case, at 2 ml/kg, for an 80 kg man and 15% burn, we require $2 \times 80 \times 15 = 2400$ ml in 24 hours. As half is given in the first 8 hours, a prescription should be made for 150 ml/hr, which equates to 1200 ml over 8 hours. Please note this calculation does not include maintenance fluid, which will be in addition to this.

Answer 28: B. Exit wounds from a gunshot will be located in a line made from the pistol and the entry wound

Bullets do not always follow a single trajectory but follow the line of least resistance. It is important to establish the path with which the bullet has taken to ascertain which anatomic structures are likely to have been involved.

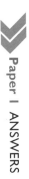

Answer 29: D. The normal cerebral blood flow in healthy adults is 20 ml/minute/100 g brain tissue

In healthy adults, cerebral blood flow is 50 ml/minute/100 g brain tissue. While the flow rate is similar in infants, it gradually increases to a peak of 90 ml/minute/100 g brain tissue at the age of 5. Brain injury can reduce cerebral blood flow for the first few hours, but this tends to normalize in the subsequent days. The cerebral perfusion pressure is calculated by the mean arterial pressure minus the intracranial pressure. A cerebral perfusion pressure between 50 and 150 mmHg is required to maintain a constant cerebral blood flow. Cerebral blood flow is reduced by hypotension, hypoxia and hypocapnia.

Answer 30: E. Surgical airway

A sucking wound is characteristic of an open pneumothorax, caused by large defects in the chest wall that remain open. An opening in the chest of more than two-thirds of the diameter of the trachea allows air to pass preferentially through the chest wound. This impairs ventilation, resulting in hypoxia, hypercarbia and respiratory acidosis. Management is initially by closing the defect with a sterile occlusive dressing that overlaps the wound and is taped on three sides. This creates a flutter valve, allowing air to escape on expiration, but avoiding air entry during inspiration. Definitive treatment is by insertion of a chest drain remote to the site of the wound.

Answer 31: C. 5%

Approximately 5% of patients with brain injury have an associated spinal injury. Conversely, 25% of spinal injury patients have an associated brain injury.

Answer 32: D. 4

The eye opening component of the GCS is as follows:

1 No response
2 Eyes open to pain
3 Eyes open to voice
4 Eyes open spontaneously

Answer 33: A. Cervical

Approximately 55% of all spinal injuries occur in the cervical region, 15% occur in the thoracic region, 15% in the thoracolumbar, and 15% in the lumbar-sacral area.

Answer 34: E. All of the above

During the primary survey, control of external haemorrhage (e.g. from fractures prior to reduction) forms part of the assessment of the circulation. The main assessment of the musculoskeletal system occurs during the secondary survey and baseline X-rays are obtained as a form of adjunct to the secondary survey.

Answer 35: E. Pedestrian versus cyclist: deceleration injury

Deceleration injuries tend to occur with high-energy accidents. They result when there is differential movement between a mobile body part and a fixed body part. Examples include the mobile aortic arch against the fixed descending aorta and the mobile lobes of the liver against the fixed ligamentum teres.

Answer 36: E. All of the above

All the listed information is of use to the receiving hospital. However, this can be communicated by telephone, fax or electronically. Documentation should not delay transfer under any circumstances.

Answer 37: D. Every 2 hours

Ideally the spinally immobilized patient should be removed from a rigid spine board and log rolled every 2 hours, to minimize the risk of developing pressure sores.

Answer 38: B. Two litres

Displaced femoral fractures can result in up to 2 litres of blood loss into the thigh, which, in the multiple injuries patient, may manifest itself as Class 3 shock. Reduction and splinting significantly decreases subsequent haemorrhage.

Answer 39: D. 36%

Assessing the extent of burns is done quickly using Wallace's 'rule of nines'. The body is fractioned into units divisible by nine, as follows:

Head and neck	9%
Upper limb	9% each
Anterior torso	18%
Posterior torso	18%
Lower limb	18% each
Perineum	1%
Total	100%

In this case: both arms = 9% + 9% and front torso = 18%, giving a total of 36%.

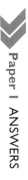

All depths of burn except first grade are included in assessing the burned area. An alternate way of assessing the extent of the burn is to use the patient's palm to represent an area of 1%. Although the 'rule of nines' is useful in adults, it is inaccurate for children due to the relative disproportionate size of certain body parts (e.g. the head is relatively larger). Most burn units have charts (e.g. the Lund & Browder chart) that can more accurately predict body surface areas with respect to age.

Answer 40: E. Around 10% of children who sustain severe multisystem trauma have residual personality changes at 1 year

As the child's skeleton is incompletely calcified, it is more pliable. Hence, internal organ damage is often seen without an overlying bony fracture. Indeed, the identification of fractures in children suggests the transfer of a massive amount of energy, and underlying organ injuries should be suspected. The body surface area to body volume ratio is higher in children (but diminishes with age), and thermal energy loss is thus a greater risk, and hypothermia can develop more quickly. As many as 60% of children suffering severe multisystem trauma have residual personality changes at 1 year after discharge, and up to 50% have either a cognitive or physical disability. Childhood injuries can have an impact on the wider family, with emotional or personality disturbances found in two-thirds of uninjured siblings. Injuries through growth plates can result in long-term growth abnormalities, such as leg-length discrepancy (femur) or scoliosis (thoracic vertebra).

Answer 41: C. Post-crash location of the patient

The pre- and post-crash location of the patient gives an idea as to whether the patient was ejected and the distance the patient was thrown. Damage to the vehicle provides a directional indication of forces applied across a fracture site. The use of a safety restraint may indicate potential spinal, intra-abdominal and C-spine injuries. If the patient fell it is important to form a mental picture of how the patient landed. If the patient was hit by a vehicle, what was the orientation of the limb during the collision? An AMPLE history is always required. This includes any allergies, the mechanism of ingestion of pharmacological or recreational drugs, psychiatric complaints and previous musculoskeletal injuries. Additional pre-hospital information includes the position in which the patient was found, the extent of bleeding at the scene (as a rule of thumb the number of units of blood that have been lost are 'blood on the floor and four more'), exposed bone ends, open wounds and any obvious deformity. In the acute trauma situation, consideration of last meal or fluid input is largely academic. If the airway is compromised, then a rapid sequence induction of anaesthesia will usually be performed.

Answer 42: A. Subcutaneous emphysema

Fracture of the larynx is rare and can present with airway obstruction. The typical triad of symptoms in laryngeal fracture is (1) hoarseness, (2) subcutaneous emphysema, and (3) a palpable fracture. Severe respiratory distress or complete airway obstruction warrants intubation (or a surgical airway if this fails). These injuries may be associated with trauma to the oesophagus, carotid artery or jugular vein. CT imaging can help confirm the diagnosis (although airway management should not be delayed!).

Distended neck veins in the trauma setting can be due to pneumothorax or pericardial effusion.

Answer 43: E. Full thickness

A first-degree burn is erythematous and painful without evidence of blistering. It is confined to the epidermis. A second-degree burn (also known as a partial thickness burn) is characteristically red and mottled with evidence of swelling and blistering. Injury extends into the dermis. A third-degree burn (full thickness) appears leathery, dry, and can be dark or waxy white. It can (but not always) be painless representing injury to the nerve endings within the subcutaneous layer.

Answer 44: B. Isolated fracture (non-long bone)

By definition the multiple-injured trauma patient has the potential for distracting injuries. Assessment of the extremities has three goals: identification of life-threatening injury, identification of limb-threatening injury and a systematic review of all musculoskeletal areas to look for any other injuries. It involves a history and rigorous examination of the bones and joints to highlight any tenderness, swelling, deformity, laxity and an assessment of the range of movement of the joints. This is then followed by assessment of the neurovascular status of all limbs. The final part of the musculoskeletal examination is baseline radiography of suspected injured areas.

Answer 45: D. Full range of motion but less than normal strength

The MRC scale for assessing muscle power is a reliable and validated scale, first published by the Medical Research Council in 1975. Each muscle group can be graded as follows:

0   Total paralysis
1   Palpable or visible contraction
2   Full range of motion with gravity eliminated
3   Full range of motion against gravity
4   Full range of motion but less than normal strength
5   Normal strength
NT Non-testable

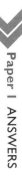

Answer 46: B. Minor

This patient's GCS is 15. He opens his eyes spontaneously (E4), can obey commands (M6) and has orientated speech (V5). This classifies the brain injury as 'minor'. The classification of brain injury is as follows: minor (GCS 13 to 15); moderate (GCS 9 to 12); and severe (GCS 3 to 8). The terms 'very minor' and 'life-threatening' do not exist in this context. A GCS of 8 or less has become an accepted definition of coma, and urgent anaesthetic input is required for airway assessment and consideration of intubation.

Answer 47: C. Two people: one person provides in-line stabilization of the head and neck, the other removes the helmet in the supine position

Trauma patients with a helmet who require airway management need the head and neck immobilized in a neutral position before helmet removal. One person therefore immobilizes the head and neck in-line from below. A second person expands the helmet laterally before gently removing it, taking care to clear the nose and occiput. Once the helmet is removed, the second person takes over in-line immobilization from above. Where possible, a cast cutter may be used to remove the helmet under immobilization, thus reducing unnecessary movement of the cervical spine. A third person is not required. Clearly, the other methods described are unsafe in the setting of a potential cervical injury.

Answer 48: E. All of the above

Pelvic disruption is associated with tears to the pelvic venous plexus and, in severe anterio-posterior compression injuries, internal iliac vessel rupture. Commonly associated injuries include genito-urinary complications.

Answer 49: E. Treatment with 100% oxygen increases the rate of dissociation of carboxyhaemoglobin

Inhalation of carbon monoxide (CO) can result in nausea and headaches, confusion, coma and death, but low-level inhalation is often asymptomatic. CO bonds to haemoglobin around 240 times as well as oxygen (to form carboxyhaemoglobin). Furthermore, dissociation is slow, with a half-life of 4 hours in room air. Treatment with 100% oxygen reduces the dissociation half-life of carboxyhaemoglobin to approximately 40 minutes. Oxygen is delivered by a non-rebreathe mask. Intubation is not routinely required. The cherry-red skin discolouration is a rare feature. Indeed, this is more commonly seen in the deceased, as the discolouration masks the usual bluish pallor.

Answer 50: B. Anterior shoulder dislocation: ulnar nerve

Although a full neurological assessment of an injured limb should be carried out, it is worthwhile considering which nerve or nerves are most likely to be affected.

Fibular neck fractures are associated with superficial peroneal nerve damage causing impairment of ankle eversion, and a sensory deficit of the lateral aspect of the dorsum of the foot.

The function of the axillary nerve and musculocutaneous nerve should be noted in anterior shoulder dislocations. From a medicolegal standpoint, this should also be documented in the notes prior to reduction on the joint. Assessing shoulder abduction and the sensation over the military badge area tests axillary nerve function. The musculocutaneous nerve can be tested by assessing elbow flexion and the sensation of the lateral aspect of the forearm.

Acetabular fractures can damage both superior and inferior gluteal nerves, which are predominantly motor nerves. Hip abduction and extension should be evaluated, respectively. Childhood supracondylar fractures can result in an absence of flexion of the middle finger distal interphalangeal joint. Dislocations of the knee can result in posterior tibial nerve palsy, leading to an absence of toe flexion and paraesthesia in the sole of the foot.

3

PAPER 2 QUESTIONS

Question 1

You attend a trauma call for a 32-year-old cyclist and suspect he has airway obstruction.
Which of the following is not an objective sign of possible airway obstruction?

A. Agitation
B. Obtundation
C. Cyanosis
D. Accessory muscle use
E. Subcutaneous emphysema

Question 2

A patient is brought in by ambulance following a motor vehicle collision and is found to have both vasodilation and relative hypovolaemia. There is no clear evidence of haemorrhage.
What type of shock are they most likely to have?

A. Cardiogenic shock
B. Neurogenic shock
C. Hypovolaemic shock
D. Addisonian shock
E. Not enough information to say

Question 3

Which of the following is not consistent with a massive haemothorax?

A. Accumulation of more than a third of the patient's blood volume in the chest cavity
B. Accumulation of over 1500 ml of blood in the chest cavity
C. Distension of the neck veins
D. Ipsilateral hyperresonance to percussion
E. Large accumulation of blood in a hemithorax resulting in respiratory compromise

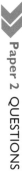

Question 4

A patient, who is opening his eyes to a voice command, is confused and localizing to painful stimuli.
What is his Glasgow Coma Score (GCS)?

A. 3
B. 6
C. 7
D. 12
E. 15

Question 5

Which of the following describes the features of central cord syndrome?

A. Left-sided neurological signs worse than the right
B. Right-sided neurological signs worse than the left
C. Upper limb neurological signs worse than the lower limbs
D. Lower limb neurological signs worse than the upper limbs
E. Ipsilateral loss of power below the lesion and contralateral loss of pain and temperature

Question 6

A 20-year-old man is brought to the emergency department with a head injury of unknown cause. On examination there is clear fluid arising from the ear and nose, and evidence of bruising behind the left ear. The patient vomits twice during the consultation.
Which of the following features does not specifically suggest an underlying basilar skull fracture?

A. Bruising behind the left ear
B. Clear fluid from the ear
C. Clear fluid from the nose
D. Vomiting
E. All of the above point specifically to a basal skull fracture

Question 7

A patient is admitted having been assaulted. As part of the surgical team you examine his abdomen. You detect percussion tenderness in the left flank. Which of the following options is not appropriate?

A. Carefully assess for rebound tenderness
B. Auscultate the abdomen to determine whether an ileus is present
C. Once your examination is complete, ensure the patient is covered knowing that hypothermia contributes to impaired coagulation
D. Examine the pelvis for stability, carefully documenting your findings
E. Inspect the gluteal region for associated injuries

Question 8

You are about to perform a rapid sequence intubation.
Which of the following is not part of the sequence?

A. Pre-oxygenate with 100% oxygen
B. Apply pressure over the thyroid cartilage
C. Administer an induction drug
D. Administer a muscle relaxant
E. Intubation

Question 9

A 42-year-old man is admitted following a road traffic collision. Although there is no evidence of penetrating trauma, the patient is hypoxic, tachycardic and hypotensive, with decreased air entry and dullness to percussion over the right hemithorax. A haemothorax is suspected and a subsequent chest drain confirms the diagnosis.
Which of the following is a poor indication for thoracotomy?

A. A persistent drain loss of over 200 ml/hour
B. Immediate drain output of over 1500 ml
C. Inability to stabilize the patient
D. Persistent need for blood transfusion
E. The presence of bright blood in the tube suggestive of an arterial source

Question 10

A 49-year-old engineer is forced to stop his car on the hard shoulder of the motorway due to a mechanical failure. As he steps out of the vehicle a passing lorry sideswipes him. He sustained multiple injuries of which the most serious is a crush amputation to the thigh.

As the first responder on scene, what is the best way to control the bleeding from his mangled limb at the roadside?

A. Elevate what is remaining of the crushed limb
B. Apply direct pressure to the thigh
C. Establish intravenous access
D. Apply a tourniquet
E. Wrap the thigh with bandages

Question 11

A 21-year-old man has just undergone a CT brain scan following a head injury. Which of the following features would suggest a subdural haematoma?

A. A biconvex lesion of an intensity suggestive of blood
B. A crescentic lesion of an intensity suggestive of blood
C. Diffuse swelling of the brain with loss of normal grey–white distinction
D. Lesions within the cerebrum of an intensity suggestive of blood
E. Petechial haemorrhages

Question 12

Central cord syndrome is classically seen in which of the following mechanisms of injury?

A. Axial compression type injuries
B. Lateral flexion type injuries
C. Hyperflexion injuries
D. Hyperextension injuries
E. Lap belt injuries

Question 13

As part of a trauma call, you are asked to see a 59-year-old gentleman who has self-harmed. He has taken a knife to his forearm and made multiple deep incisions. This is not the first time that he has self-harmed in this way. As part of your assessment, you see that the lacerations extend deep to the investing fascia. You are unable to palpate an ulnar pulse and there is demonstrable motor and sensory deficit in an ulnar nerve distribution. The capillary refill time distally is 2 seconds. His pulse is 120/min and blood pressure is 80/55 mmHg.
What is your next course of action?

A. Ascertain whether an ulnar pulse is detectable with a handheld Doppler probe
B. Check his old notes to see if his neurovascular deficit is pre-existing
C. Commence an intravenous fluid infusion
D. Explore the wounds under local anaesthesia to ascertain whether the ulna artery has been lacerated
E. Refer to your local plastic surgery team in light of the neurovascular deficit

Question 14

You are the first responder to a 17-year-old girl who has been stabbed in the anterior chest wall on the left-hand side. On examination she is in extremis. You find there is tracheal deviation to the right and there is hyperresonance and quiet breath sounds throughout the left side.
What should you do?

A. Tube thoracostomy at fifth intercostal space, anterior to the mid-axillary line, left-hand side
B. Tube thoracostomy at fifth intercostal space, anterior to the mid-axillary line, right-hand side
C. Needle decompression at second intercostal space mid-axillary line, left-hand side
D. Needle decompression at second intercostal space mid-clavicular line, right-hand side
E. Needle decompression at second intercostal space mid-clavicular line, left-hand side

Question 15

Which of the following is not a feature consistent with cardiac tamponade?

A. A rise in jugular venous pressure on inspiration
B. Clearly defined gallop rhythm on auscultation
C. Hypotension
D. Pulseless electrical activity
E. Raised jugular venous pressure

Question 16

A 34-year-old woman is admitted to the hospital within half an hour of a head injury.
Which of the following is an indication for a CT brain scan?

A. A deep skull laceration
B. A single reported episode of vomiting since the injury
C. Age of 34
D. Amnesia of an hour prior to the injury
E. GCS of 14 on admission

Question 17

Which of the following statements regarding anterior cord syndrome is TRUE?

A. There is loss of posterior column function
B. Classically affects the upper limbs more than the lower limbs
C. Has the best prognosis of incomplete injuries
D. Is characterized by paraplegia and loss of pain and temperature sensation
E. Is usually caused by a hyperextension injury

Question 18

The radial nerve in the upper limb provides innervation to all except which of the following?

A. Triceps brachii
B. Flexor pollicis brevis
C. Extensor digitorum communis
D. Sensation in the first dorsal web space
E. Extensor carpi radialis

Question 19

An 18-month-old boy is brought into the emergency department by his parents. He was lowered into a bath of water that was too hot and sustained burns to the full length of both his legs on the posterior aspect and also his buttocks.
Estimate the percentage burn he has sustained.

A. 9%
B. 14%
C. 19%
D. 32%
E. 40%

Question 20

You are asked to perform an airway maintenance manoeuvre during a trauma call while awaiting the arrival of an anaesthetist.
Which of the following statements about these manoeuvres is FALSE?

A. The chin should be lifted anteriorly in the chin lift
B. The neck needs to be hyperextended in the chin lift and the jaw thrust
C. It is appropriate to rest the hands on the maxilla during the jaw thrust
D. If simple airway-opening manoeuvres fail, an oropharyngeal or nasopharyngeal airway may be of benefit
E. Immobilization of the cervical spine is essential during these procedures

Question 21

The femoral nerve is involved in which one of the following?

A. Knee extension
B. Knee flexion
C. Sensation to the outer aspect of the thigh
D. Great toe dorsiflexion
E. Sensation to the sole of the foot

Question 22

Which of the following terms is used to describe a burst fracture of the first cervical vertebra?

A. Jefferson fracture
B. Hangman's fracture
C. Greater compression fracture
D. Chance fracture
E. Wedge compression fracture

Question 23

A 28-year-old man is admitted to the emergency department following a stabbing. On examination he is tachycardic and hypotensive, with distended neck veins and an obvious wound to the left side of his chest. Air entry is normal and the chest is resonant to percussion.
Which of the following is the definitive management for the likely underlying condition?

A. Chest drain insertion
B. Intubation and positive pressure ventilation
C. Needle thoracocentesis
D. Pericardiocentesis
E. Pericardiotomy

Question 24

Which of the following is TRUE regarding hypovolaemic shock?

A. Class 1 shock is associated with a urine output greater than 30 ml/hour, a respiratory rate of 14–20 breaths per minute and a decreased pulse pressure
B. Class 2 shock is associated with 750–1500 ml of blood loss, a raised respiratory rate of 20–30 breaths per minute and a urine output of 20–30 ml/hour
C. Class 4 haemorrhage represents the smallest volume of blood loss that is consistently associated with a drop in systolic blood pressure
D. Class 3 shock is associated with a lowered urine output of 5–15 ml/hour and a pulse of 100–120/min
E. Class 4 shock is associated with >2000 ml of blood loss and an increase in pulse pressure

Question 25

In which of the following positions is it safest to immobilize the hand and wrist?

A. Full flexion
B. Edinburgh position
C. Dublin position
D. Full extension
E. Straight

Question 26

Which of the following statements regarding chemical burns is NOT true?

A. Alkali burns are more serious than acid ones
B. Antibiotics are not indicated
C. If dry powder is present, this should be brushed away before washing is commenced
D. Neutralizing agents should be used
E. The affected area should be washed with water

Question 27

Regarding the surgical management of head injuries, which of the following statements is NOT true?

A. Depressed skull fractures need operative elevation if the degree of depression is half the thickness of the adjacent skull
B. Intracranial mass lesions should be treated by a neurosurgeon
C. Penetrating injuries require monitoring of the intracranial pressure
D. Prophylactic antibiotics are given for penetrating injuries
E. Scalp wounds without underlying fractures can be closed safely

Question 28

In which of the following scenarios would diagnostic peritoneal lavage NOT be indicated?

A. A patient with a penetrating abdominal injury who is haemodynamically unstable
B. A patient who fell from a roof, who is now tachycardic and complaining of altered sensation
C. A patient who is haemodynamically normal but no FAST scan or abdominal CT is available
D. A pedestrian who has collided with a four-wheel-drive vehicle is haemodynamically unstable and has fractured his pelvis
E. A front seat passenger in a car is involved in a high-speed impact; he is confused and disorientated but complaining of abdominal pain

Question 29

A patient who was recently admitted to an emergency department requires urgent transfer to a tertiary centre.
Which of the following investigations must be completed prior to transfer?

A. C-spine X-rays
B. Haemoglobin
C. ECG
D. Oxygen saturations
E. None of the above

Question 30

A 31-year-old man has sustained an injury to the chest and is brought into the emergency room. He is being assessed for signs of life in the presence of a qualified cardiac surgeon.
Which of the following features suggests he is a candidate for resuscitative thoracotomy?

A. Blunt injury with a feeble pulse and no signs of life
B. Blunt injury with pulseless electrical activity and signs of life
C. Penetrating injury with a feeble pulse and signs of life
D. Penetrating injury with pulseless electrical activity and no signs of life
E. Penetrating injury with pulseless electrical activity and signs of life

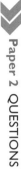

Question 31

You are called to assess the airway of a multiple-injured patient.
Which one of the following Glasgow Coma Scores would suggest the need for prompt intubation?

A. 15
B. 13
C. 11
D. 9
E. 7

Question 32

With regard to the anatomy of the brain and skull, which of the following statements is FALSE?

A. The meningeal arteries are located between the dura and the skull
B. Epidural haematomas often lead to a rapid increase in intracranial pressure
C. The pterion is an anatomical weak spot of the skull under which the anterior branch of the middle meningeal artery lies
D. The subdural space exists because the arachnoid membrane is not adhered to the dura
E. The pia mater is attached to the arachnoid membrane

Question 33

The inability to flex the elbow indicates injury to which of the following nerve roots?

A. C5 and C6
B. C6 and C7
C. C7
D. C8
E. T1

Question 34

A 45-year-old Jehovah's Witness has fallen from a horse. She has an open-book fracture of her pelvis and a GCS of 13. She is tachycardic and hypotensive despite intravenous fluids. Her partner insists that she has a strongly held belief that she should not have any blood transfusion. She has refused blood transfusions in the past.
What should you do?

A. Proceed with a blood transfusion despite her partner's concerns
B. Consider other blood products such as fresh frozen plasma (FFP)
C. Continue with a further crystalloid infusion
D. Apply a pelvic binder and consider urgent embolization
E. Tell the partner that, as the patient has an altered conscious level, this decision is to be made by the doctors looking after her

Question 35

Regarding the airway management in paediatric trauma, which of the following statements is TRUE?

A. An infant's trachea is approximately 8 cm long
B. An oropharyngeal airway should be inserted backwards and rotated 180 degrees into position
C. Intubation should be performed with cuffed tubes in younger children
D. The optimum position for airway opening is with the face parallel to the plane of the bed
E. Pre-oxygenation is not required before intubation

Question 36

A 45-year-old female is admitted 30 minutes after having had a high-speed road traffic accident. On examination of her abdomen, you see a prominent lap belt sign. You suspect a small bowel injury.
What would be the most effective imaging modality to confirm this suspicion?

A. CT abdomen
B. Diagnostic peritoneal lavage
C. Ultrasound scan
D. Abdominal radiograph
E. MRI abdomen

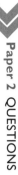

Question 37

A sensory level at the umbilicus indicates spinal involvement to the level of which of the following?

A. T1
B. T4
C. T6
D. T8
E. T10

Question 38

Which of the following is most accurate at predicting mortality in geriatric trauma?

A. Metabolic alkalosis
B. Metabolic acidosis
C. Respiratory alkalosis
D. Respiratory acidosis
E. $PaCO_2$

Question 39

There are numerous changes that occur during pregnancy. Having an appreciation of these changes is imperative in treating trauma in females.
Which of the following statements best describes the growth of the foetus?

A. The uterus expands in size, emerging from the pelvic brim by week 10
B. The mother's abdominal viscera are pushed posteriorly to make room for the foetus
C. The uterus is thicker-walled in trimester 3 in comparison to trimester 2
D. Foetal skull fractures late in pregnancy can result from a mother's pelvic fracture
E. The placenta is highly elastic

Question 40

You are preparing a tray of drugs in readiness for a rapid sequence intubation. Which one of the following statements about relevant drugs is correct?

A. Etomidate has a marked effect on both blood pressure and intracranial pressure
B. Succinylcholine has a rapid onset and is long-acting
C. Flumazenil may be used to reverse the effects of benzodiazepines
D. Succinylcholine administrations carry a risk of hypokalaemia
E. Sedative drugs should be avoided in rapid sequence intubation

Question 41

Assessment of sensation provided by the radial nerve is performed by touching which of the following?

A. Fifth finger
B. First web space
C. Fingertips
D. Regimental patch area
E. Armpit

Question 42

Which of the following statements is TRUE regarding trauma in elderly patients?

A. Patients on long-term diuretics are likely to have a chronically contracted intravascular volume
B. BP >120 mmHg suggests a normal circulating volume
C. Once corrected for their smaller lean body mass, the fluid requirements of elderly patients are less than that of younger patients
D. Patients on long-term diuretics are likely to have a metabolic acidosis
E. Fluid resuscitation of the elderly patient should be more aggressive, due to likely increases in systemic vascular resistance and cardiac afterload

Question 43

What is the likelihood of a patient with a traumatic brain injury having an associated spinal injury?

A. 1%
B. 2%
C. 5%
D. 25%
E. 55%

Question 44

An inappropriate response to questions scores how many points on the GCS?

A. 1
B. 2
C. 3
D. 4
E. 5

Question 45

At which level does the spinal cord terminate?

A. T11
B. T12
C. L1
D. L2
E. L3

Question 46

A 28-year-old homeless man presents to the emergency department during a particularly cold winter evening. He complains of pain in his left foot. On examination there is hyperaemia and oedema of the great toe without evidence of skin necrosis. Warming of the foot does not improve the clinical picture. Which of the following is the likely diagnosis?

A. Gangrene
B. Frostbite, first degree
C. Frostbite, second degree
D. Frostbite, third degree
E. Frostnip

Question 47

A 4-year-old child has fallen from a staircase. He has suffered multiple injuries but remains conscious.
Given that he has a partially obstructed airway, how should the patient be managed?

A. Jaw thrust manoeuvre with bimanual in-line stabilization, without raising the body
B. Raise the body of the child by placing him on a pad such that the face is parallel to the floor
C. Jaw thrust, bimanual in-line stabilization and raise the body
D. Insert a nasopharyngeal tube
E. Insert an oropharyngeal tube

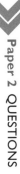

Question 48

A 67-year-old woman of no fixed abode presents to the emergency department after sleeping rough for three nights over the winter period. She complains of cold hands, which are painful. On examination three digits of the right hand are hyperaemic and there is evidence of skin necrosis.
Which of the following is not part of an appropriate management plan?

A. Analgesia
B. Check tetanus status
C. Elevate the hands
D. Place the hands under a dry heat source
E. Warm fluids by mouth

Question 49

How many people are required to perform a log roll?

A. Three people
B. Four people
C. Five people
D. Six people
E. Seven people

Question 50

What morphology of brain injury would a laceration to the sagittal dural sinus result in?

A. Extradural haematoma
B. Subdural haematoma
C. Intracerebral haemorrhage
D. Diffuse brain injury
E. Petechial haemorrhages

4

Answer 1: E. Subcutaneous emphysema

There are several objective signs of airway obstruction. Agitation can result from hypoxia, and hypercarbia can cause obtundation. Cyanosis can be observed in the nail beds and circumoral skin, and indicates hypoxaemia secondary to inadequate ventilation. Accessory muscles are employed in an attempt to improve ventilation in the setting of airway compromise. Other objective features of airway obstruction include noisy breathing (for example, snoring or stridor with partial occlusion of the pharynx/larynx) or dysphonia (hoarseness) with laryngeal obstruction.

Subcutaneous emphysema describes the presence of air within the subcutaneous tissues. It usually occurs on the chest, neck and face, where it travels along the fascial planes. Subcutaneous emphysema can result from blunt or penetrating chest trauma, pneumothorax or pneumomediastinum. Trauma to the upper airway, for example, laryngeal fracture, can also result in this feature.

Answer 2: B. Neurogenic shock

The majority of shock in trauma is caused by hypovolaemia. However, this clinical scenario describes something different. Neurogenic shock presents with both vasodilation and relative hypovolaemia. Spinal cord injury may produce hypotension as a result of insufficient sympathetic tone. Patients will be unable to mount a tachycardia or prevent cutaneous vasodilatation. In patients that do not respond to aggressive fluid therapy, consider ongoing haemorrhage or neurogenic shock.

Answer 3: D. Ipsilateral hyperresonance to percussion

A massive haemothorax results from the rapid accumulation of more than 1500 ml of blood (or more than a third of the patient's circulating blood volume) in the chest cavity. It most often occurs secondary to penetrating injuries disrupting the systemic or hilar vessels. Features include ipsilateral absent breath sounds and dullness to percussion. Although the neck veins are characteristically flat (due to hypovolaemia), they may rarely be distended if there is an associated mediastinal shift.

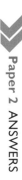

Answer 4: D. 12

This patient opens his eyes to a voice command (3), is confused (4) and localizes to painful stimuli (5), giving a GCS of 12.

Answer 5: C. Upper limb neurological signs worse than the lower limbs

Central cord syndrome is the most common spinal cord lesion. It occurs in older people with cervical spondylosis who sustain a hyperextension injury. There is a flaccid weakness of the arms, but motor and sensory fibres to the lower limb are comparatively preserved, as these are located more peripherally in the spinal cord. There is a varying degree of sensory loss. Central cord lesions have a fair prognosis.

Answer 6: D. Vomiting

Signs of basilar skull fractures include CSF otorrhoea, CSF rhinorrhoea, Battle's sign (bruising by the mastoid process), haemotympanum, raccoon eyes (periorbital ecchymoses) and cranial nerve palsies (often VII and VIII, which may occur a few days after the initial injury). Vomiting can occur from a head injury of any cause and does not specifically relate to a basilar skull fracture.

Answer 7: A. Carefully assess for rebound tenderness

In this situation there is no need to ascertain whether rebound tenderness is present. By doing so, the patient will be subjected to unnecessary pain. The fact that there are signs of peritonism mandates the need for further investigation.

Answer 8: B. Apply pressure over the thyroid cartilage

The technique described for rapid sequence intubation (RSI) in the ATLS manual is as follows: pre-oxygenate with 100% oxygen; apply pressure over the cricoid cartilage (not the thyroid cartilage); administer, as induction drug or sedation, succinylcholine (a.k.a. suxamethonium, a quick-acting and short-acting muscle relaxant); intubate orotracheally; inflate cuff and confirm placement; release cricoid pressure and ventilate patient.

Answer 9: E. The presence of bright blood in the tube suggestive of an arterial source

The decision for a thoracotomy in the context of massive haemothorax should be made by a qualified surgeon. Indications for thoracotomy include an immediate drain output of over 1500 ml, a persistent high drain loss of blood, a persistent need for transfusion and an inability to stabilize the patient. The colour of the blood, suggesting an arterial or venous source, is a poor indicator of the necessity for thoracotomy. A thoracotomy is not indicated unless a qualified surgeon is present.

Answer 10: D. Apply a tourniquet

In this scenario, the patient will undoubtedly develop life-threatening shock if not treated quickly. Rapid haemorrhage control must be achieved. Application of a tourniquet high on the proximal thigh is likely to be the most effective method of preventing further bleeding until it can be definitively managed in the hospital setting. Although establishing intravenous access is obviously of critical importance, it will do nothing to control the bleeding, which is what the question asks.

Answer 11: B. A crescentic lesion of an intensity suggestive of blood

The CT brain scan of a subdural haematoma typically results in a crescentic haematoma between the brain and the skull. A biconvex haematoma in the same region occurs with an epidural haematoma. Intracerebral haemorrhages occur within the cerebrum. Diffuse brain injury can result in a global swelling with loss of the normal grey–white distinction. Another diffuse pattern, often seen in high-velocity impacts or deceleration injuries, may produce multiple punctate haemorrhages.

Answer 12: D. Hyperextension injuries

Central cord syndrome commonly follows a forward fall directly onto the face, causing hyperextension. Associated findings often include a forehead laceration or bruising.

With forced hyperextension there is reduced space available for the cord leading to localized trauma.

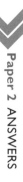

Answer 13: C. Commence an intravenous fluid infusion

It is imperative to realize the seriousness of this patient's injuries. The first thing to note is that the gentleman is in at least class 3 shock and will have lost a minimum of 30% of his circulating volume. His haemodynamic instability must be addressed immediately. Due to this level of shock, it can be assumed with confidence that a significant vascular injury has occurred if this is an isolated injury.

Answer 14: E. Needle decompression at second intercostal space mid-clavicular line, left-hand side

This patient has a left-sided tension pneumothorax. Without immediate treatment she is likely to die. A needle decompression (thoracentesis) at the second intercostal space in the mid-clavicular line will convert this tension pneumothorax to a simple pneumothorax. The definitive management is a chest drain (tube thoracostomy), but this can be performed once the primary survey is complete.

Answer 15: B. Clearly defined gallop rhythm on auscultation

Cardiac tamponade most commonly occurs after penetrating injuries, although blunt trauma can be the offending cause. Features of cardiac tamponade include Beck's triad (raised jugular venous pressure [JVP], muffled heart sounds and hypotension), Kussmaul's sign (a rise in JVP on inspiration) and pulseless electrical activity.

Claude Schaeffer Beck, American cardiac surgeon (1894–1971)
Adolph Kussmaul, German physician (1822–1902)

Answer 16: D. Amnesia of an hour prior to the injury

Indications for a CT brain scan following a head injury include: a GCS <15 after the immediate 2 hours following the injury, an open/depressed or suspected basal skull fracture, two separate episodes of vomiting, age over 65 years, amnesia of over 30 minutes prior to the injury, focal neurological deficit and seizures. If a CT scan following a head injury is normal, the patient can return home with written advice, assuming they can be observed for 24 hours and that there is no evidence of drug or alcohol intoxication.

Answer 17: D. Is characterized by paraplegia and loss of pain and temperature sensation

The anterior cord syndrome occurs secondary to a flexion-compression injury. There is loss of neurological function of the anterior two-thirds of the spinal cord, namely, the spinothalamic (pain and temperature) and corticospinal (motor) tracts. There is greater motor loss in the legs than the arms. Dorsal column function is usually preserved. The anterior cord syndrome has the worst prognosis of all spinal cord lesions.

Answer 18: B. Flexor pollicis brevis

The radial nerve provides nerve supply to the wrist extensors, elbow extensors and sensation to the first dorsal web space. Flexor pollicis brevis is innervated by the median nerve.

Answer 19: C. 19%

The adult 'rule of nines' must be adapted for use in children on account of the disproportionate size of the head, torso and limbs. Thus, this aide memoir in paediatrics should follow:

Head	18%
Anterior torso	18%
Back	13%
Buttocks	5%
Upper limbs	4.5% for each anterior and posterior aspects
Lower limbs	7% for each anterior and posterior aspects

In this case: 7% + 7% + 5% = 19%

Answer 20: B. The neck needs to be hyperextended in the chin lift and jaw thrust

In the setting of decreased consciousness, the tongue can flop posteriorly and obstruct the hypopharynx. This is easily corrected by either the chin-lift or jaw-thrust manoeuvres. As both of these may aggravate C-spine injury, in-line immobilization is essential. In the chin lift, the fingers of one hand are placed under the mandible and the chin lifted anteriorly. The ipsilateral thumb can be used to depress the lower lip and keep the mouth open. In the jaw thrust, the angles of the jaw are grasped while resting the hand on the maxilla and the mandible displaced forward. The neck should not be hyperextended during either of these manoeuvres, as this risks converting a cervical fracture without cord injury into one with cord injury. If simple airway manoeuvres fail, oropharyngeal or nasopharyngeal airways may be useful.

Answer 21: A. Knee extension

The femoral nerve (L2,3,4) supplies knee extension and sensation to the inner thigh, and is commonly associated with pubic rami fractures. Knee flexion is provided by the sciatic nerve and great toe dorsiflexion is provided by the peroneal nerve. Sensation to the outer aspect of the thigh is from the lateral femoral cutaneous nerve, and the sole of the foot is innervated by the medial plantar nerve.

Answer 22: A. Jefferson fracture

Following axial loading there is disruption of the ring of C1 both anteriorly and posteriorly with lateral displacement of the lateral masses. During the primary survey this fracture can be seen on the 'open mouth' AP radiograph with lateral displacement of the lateral masses of C1 beside the odontoid peg.

Geoffrey Jefferson, British neurosurgeon (1886–1961)

Answer 23: E. Pericardiotomy

The clinical features in this case are consistent with a cardiac tamponade. Note the question here asks for the definitive management. The ideal management here is by operative drainage of the pericardial sac (pericardiotomy). If this is not available, a needle pericardiocentesis is a diagnostic as well as a possible therapeutic option (unless the blood in the pericardial sac has clotted). In any case, once pericardiocentesis has been performed, preparations should be made for exploratory surgery to examine the heart and repair the underlying injury.

Answer 24: B. Class 2 shock is associated with 750–1500 ml of blood loss, a raised respiratory rate of 20–30 breaths per minute and a urine output of 20–30 ml/hour

Virtually all trauma victims who have signs of shock will be treated as if they are hypovolaemic, but care should be taken to identify the small minority of patients who do have non-haemorrhagic shock. This system of categorizing haemorrhagic shock into one of four classes is based on the patient's initial presentation and can be used to estimate the volume of blood loss. A normal or increased pulse pressure is only seen in patients who have lost less than 15% of their blood volume. If the patient continues to haemorrhage, circulating catecholamines act to increase the peripheral vascular resistance. At this stage the patient will have moved from class 1 to class 2 shock. A useful aide memoire is to think of the scoring system of a game of tennis:

Class 1 hypovolaemic shock	Love: 15	0–15% blood loss
Class 2 hypovolaemic shock	15: 30	15–30% blood loss
Class 3 hypovolaemic shock	30: 40	30–40% blood loss
Class 4 hypovolaemic shock	40: game	>40% blood loss

It may be useful to memorize the following table:

	Class 1	Class 2	Class 3	Class 4
Fluid loss	<15%; <750 mL	15–30%; 750–1500 mL	30–40%; 1500–2000 mL	>40%; >2000 mL
Heart rate (bpm)	<100	100–120	120–140	>140
Blood pressure	Normal	Normal, reduced pulse pressure	Low	Very low
Respiratory rate (breaths/min)	Normal (<20)	Slightly raised (20–30)	Tachypnoeic (30–40)	Very tachypnoeic (>40)
Urine output (mL/h)	>30	20–30	10–20	<10
Mental status	Alert	Anxious	Drowsy	Confused/ unconscious

Answer 25: B. Edinburgh position

The Edinburgh position is 30 degrees of wrist extension, 90 degrees of metacarpophalangeal flexion and straight interphalangeal joints (IPJs). This helps to prevent stiffness and contractures at the metacarpophalangeal joint (MCPJ) and IPJs by holding the ligaments at maximal excursion.

Answer 26: D. Neutralizing agents should be used

Alkali burns are generally more serious than acid burns, as alkalis penetrate more deeply. The severity of a burn is influenced by the amount and concentration of the culprit agent, as well as the duration of contact. The area should immediately be washed with large amounts of water for at least 20–30 minutes, with a shower or hose if available. Dry powder should be brushed away before irrigation. Neutralizing agents offer no advantage as the neutralization reaction may produce heat, which exacerbates the injury. Antibiotics are not indicated prophylactically in any burns and are reserved for treating infection.

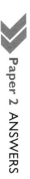

Answer 27: A. Depressed skull fractures need operative elevation if the degree of depression is half the thickness of the adjacent skull

Scalp wounds should be cleaned and, if there is no evidence of an underlying fracture, these should be closed primarily. Depressed skull fractures need operative elevation if the degree of depression is greater than the thickness of the adjacent skull, or if the fracture is open or comminuted. Intracranial mass lesions should be treated by a neurosurgeon. Penetrating injuries require CT scan assessment, along with angiography if a vascular injury is suspected. Intracranial pressure monitoring is also required as well as prophylactic antibiotics.

Answer 28: A. A patient with a penetrating abdominal injury who is haemodynamically unstable

Diagnostic peritoneal lavage is used in haemodynamically unstable patients who have sustained blunt injuries (unless CT or ultrasound scan [USS] are available). Warmed fluid is added to the abdominal cavity, mixed (performed by log rolling the patient or palpating the abdomen) and then removed for analysis. Should blood or bowel contents be aspirated, patients should undergo laparotomy.

Answer 29: E. None of the above

Following the primary survey and appropriate associated interventions, no further tests are mandatory prior to transfer.

Answer 30: E. Penetrating injury with pulseless electrical activity and signs of life

In hypovolaemic patients with cardiac arrest or pulseless electrical activity (PEA), closed heart massage is ineffective. Patients with penetrating thoracic injuries with PEA are candidates for immediate resuscitative thoracotomy, if a qualified surgeon is present at the time of the patient's arrival. Signs of life must be present, such as reactive pupils or spontaneous movement. Therapeutic manoeuvres that can be accomplished with a resuscitative thoracotomy include: evacuation of pericardial blood that is causing tamponade, direct control of intrathoracic haemorrhage, open cardiac massage, and cross-clamping of the descending aorta to improve perfusion of the brain and heart.

Answer 31: E. 7

The patient who has a Glasgow Coma Score (GCS) of 8 or less usually requires prompt intubation. However, there are many other indications for a definitive airway (e.g. apnoea, protection from aspiration, impending airway compromise) and thus a GCS above 8 does not necessarily mean intubation can be avoided.

Answer 32: E. The pia mater is attached to the arachnoid membrane

The pia mater is a thin membrane attached to the surface of the brain, not the arachnoid. Between the pia and the arachnoid flows cerebral spinal fluid (CSF), which, among other roles, acts to cushion the brain from injury. Leakage of CSF must always be looked for as part of the secondary survey. It is known as otorrhoea or rhinorrhoea if it passes from the external auditory canal or nose respectively.

Answer 33: A. C5 and C6

As a rule of thumb: the biceps is innervated by C5, C6; wrist extensors by C6; triceps by C7; wrist and finger flexors by C8; and the small muscles of the hand by T1.

Answer 34: D. Apply a pelvic binder and consider urgent embolization

This patient is in at least grade 3 shock. Her failure to respond to intravenous fluids suggests ongoing haemorrhage from the pelvis. A pelvic binder should be applied to tamponade the bleeding and consideration be made towards urgent embolization. Of note, the autonomy of Jehovah's Witnesses should be respected. It is useful, however, to clarify when possible whether other blood products are acceptable to their beliefs should the need arise.

Answer 35: D. The optimum position for airway opening is with the face parallel to the plane of the bed

The infant's trachea is around 5 cm long, and grows to 7 cm by 18 months. Failure to appreciate the short length may result in intubation of the right mainstem bronchus and inadequate ventilation. Oral airways should only be inserted if a child is unconscious (to prevent vomiting induced by the gag reflex). Such airways should be inserted directly in the correct orientation, as the rotation method used in adults risks trauma to the soft tissues of the oropharynx with resulting haemorrhage. Orotracheal intubation should be performed with uncuffed tubes in children under the age of 9 years; the cricoid ring itself forms a natural seal around the tube. The cuffs of the tube may cause oedema, ulceration or disruption of a young child's fragile airway. The airway should be optimized by keeping the plane of the face parallel to the plane of the bed or stretcher. The chin-lift position may obstruct the airway. Before any attempts to establish a mechanical airway, the child should be pre-oxygenated.

Answer 36: B. Diagnostic peritoneal lavage

Torn intra-abdominal organs can give rise to subtle signs on physical examination. Always have a high index of suspicion when linear ecchymoses or Chance fractures (flexion injury of the spine) are present. If such a tear results in a slow rate of bleeding, neither FAST nor CT scanning will be sufficiently sensitive to detect this in an early presentation. Diagnostic peritoneal lavage will.

GQ Chance, 20th century British radiologist

Answer 37: E. T10

The sensory level of the umbilicus is at T10, the nipple at T4 and the xiphisternum at T6.

Answer 38: B. Metabolic acidosis

Metabolic acidosis is a predictor of mortality. With age, cardiac index falls, circulating blood volume declines and circulation time increases. These factors predispose tissues to impaired perfusion, lactic acidosis and deranged pH. The aged kidney is also more susceptible to injury from hypoperfusion and is less able to excrete H^+ ions and normalize pH.

Answer 39: D. Foetal skull fractures late in pregnancy can result from a mother's pelvic fracture

The uterus is considered an intrapelvic organ up to 12 weeks of gestation. The uterus reaches the umbilicus by 20 weeks and the costal margin by 34 weeks. It displaces the mobile abdominal viscera vertically. As a result, penetrating injuries to the upper abdomen can cause complicated injuries to both thoracic and abdominal viscera. The thickness of the uterine wall diminishes throughout pregnancy. When the foetal head engages the pelvis in the final few weeks, it has further protection from injury from the maternal pelvis. However, should a pelvic fracture of the mother occur, the foetus is susceptible to intracranial injury. The lack of elastic tissue within the placenta can cause abruptio-placentae should a shearing force be applied.

Answer 40: C. Flumazenil may be used to reverse the effects of benzodiazepines

Etomidate, an induction drug, has little effect on blood pressure and intracranial pressure, although it can depress adrenal function. Induction agents and sedatives (including benzodiazepines) are appropriate to use, but must be used with care in the hypovolaemic patient to avoid loss of the airway as the patient becomes sedated. If benzodiazepines are used, flumazenil must be available to reverse the effects if required. Succinylcholine induces paralysis rapidly (<1 minute) and lasts up to 5 minutes only (short-acting). The reason for the short-acting agent is that if intubation is unsuccessful, the patient must be manually ventilated until paralysis resolves. Succinylcholine use increases the risk of hyperkalaemia and is therefore avoided in patients with crush injury, major burns, pre-existing chronic renal impairment and chronic neuromuscular disease.

Answer 41: B. First web space

The classical area for loss of sensation with a radial nerve palsy is the first web space. The regimental patch sign is loss of sensation over the deltoid region of the shoulder, corresponding to the area of sensation supplied by the axillary nerve.

Answer 42: A. Patients on long-term diuretics are likely to have a chronically contracted intravascular volume

The reduction in physiological reserve and co-morbidities of elderly patients creates additional challenges in managing trauma. An apparently 'normotensive' patient may be in a state of considerable hypoperfusion, having usually kept a blood pressure well above the normal range. Patients may also be 'beta blocked' and unable to mount an appropriate tachycardia.

Loop and thiazide diuretic therapy cause a contraction of the intravascular volume and commonly result in hypokalaemia and a compensated metabolic alkalosis. Once corrected for a leaner body mass, patients will require similar volumes to those of younger individuals.

Answer 43: C. 5%

Approximately 5% of patients with brain injury have an associated spinal injury. Conversely, 25% of spinal injury patients have an associated brain injury.

Answer 44: C. 3

Inappropriate responses to questions scores 3 on the GCS. The vocal component of the GCS is as follows:

1 No response
2 Incomprehensible sounds
3 Inappropriate responses
4 Confused speech
5 Appropriate speech

Answer 45: C. LI

The spinal cord terminates at the conus medullaris at the level of L1. Injuries at this level result in bladder and bowel dysfunction. Examination findings for lesions situated above this level would reveal an upper motor neuron pattern, with a lower motor neuron pattern for those below.

Answer 46: B. Frostbite, first degree

Frostbite is caused by tissue freezing with intracellular ice crystal formation, microvascular occlusions and tissue anoxia. This patient has first-degree frostbite, characterized by hyperaemia and oedema without skin necrosis. The other stages of frostbite are:

- Second degree: vesicle formation with hyperaemia/oedema and partial skin necrosis
- Third degree: full-thickness skin necrosis with haemorrhagic vesicle formation
- Fourth degree: full-thickness necrosis including muscle and bone with gangrene

Frostnip is a mild cold-induced injury associated with pain, pallor and numbness in the affected area, which reverses with warming.

Answer 47: C. Jaw thrust, bimanual in-line stabilization and raise the body

A child's cranium is disproportionately large and, when lying supine, the cervical spine is slightly flexed, which can further impede the airway. By placing the child on a mat of several blankets, the neck can be very slightly extended (in-line) enabling the airway to open further. Nasopharyngeal tubes should not be used on children aged below 9 years due to the risk of damaging the adenoids or penetrating the cranial vault. No airway adjunct should be used in a conscious patient due to a highly sensitive gag reflex and the high risk of vomiting.

Answer 48: D. Place the hands under a dry heat source

The management of cold injuries includes warm clothing and warm fluids by mouth. Injured areas should be placed in warm water (40°C) until pink (may take 20–30 minutes). Dry heat should be avoided, as should rubbing the affected area.

Patients should be given adequate analgesia. The local wound care of frostbite includes elevating the area, keeping it clean and exposed, and avoiding pressure or weight bearing. Tetanus status should be confirmed. Antibiotics are only required if there is evidence of infection. There is no role for heparin, hyperbaric oxygen therapy, vasodilators or sympathetic blockade.

Answer 49: B. Four people

Four people are needed to perform a safe log roll: one to maintain manual in-line immobilization of the head and neck; one for the torso; one for the pelvis and legs; and one to direct the procedure and remove the spine board.

Answer 50: A. Extradural haematoma

The falx cerebri is an extension of the dura mater that separates the two cerebral hemispheres. At its superior end, the dura splits into two layers, within which lies the sagittal dural sinus. A laceration to this structure would therefore result in an extradural haematoma. Of note, extradural haematomas can also result from bleeding skull fractures.

5

PAPER 3 QUESTIONS

Question 1

You are inserting a gum elastic bougie as part of a difficult intubation.
What indicators can you use to ensure you are in the trachea and not the oesophagus?

A. The clicks of the tracheal rings are felt as the tip of the bougie passes over them
B. The bougie will not pass the 20 cm mark
C. The bougie will not pass the 40 cm mark
D. The endotracheal tube passes easily over the bougie
E. There is no rotation of the tube if it passes into a main bronchus

Question 2

An elderly patient has been involved in a motor vehicle collision.
Which of the following is NOT true in consideration of trauma and the elderly population?

A. Elderly patients have an impaired ability to increase heart rate or efficiency of myocardial contraction to hypovolaemia
B. Elderly patients are less able to meet the increased demands of gas exchange caused by trauma as a result of decreased diffusion capacity and reduction in pulmonary compliance
C. Vital organs are less sensitive to reduced blood flow
D. The hormones vasopressin, cortisol and aldosterone have reduced efficacy
E. The effect of age results in a reduction of catecholamine receptors in respect to the cardiovascular system

Question 3

A 62-year-old man is brought into the local minor injuries unit following a road traffic collision. He has shortness of breath and pain to the left side of his chest. Observations include: saturations 88% on air, respiratory rate 28/minute and heart rate 96/minute. There are decreased breath sounds over the left hemithorax but the trachea is central, the neck veins are not distended and the heart sounds are normal. No penetrating injury is apparent. A chest X-ray shows a rim of air around the left lung. It is decided he needs to be transferred to a secondary care hospital. Which of the following is the most appropriate initial management option?

A. Chest drain insertion
B. Immediate transfer via air ambulance
C. Intubation and positive pressure ventilation
D. Needle thoracocentesis
E. Observation alone

Question 4

Which of the following features seen on a skull X-ray should be considered a normal finding in a 63-year-old patient who has sustained a head injury?

A. Calcification of the pineal gland
B. Hair-on-end appearance
C. Depressed skull fracture
D. Air-fluid levels in the paranasal sinuses
E. Pepper pot skull

Question 5

You are working in an emergency department. A paramedic crew brings a patient into the department on a wheelchair. He was involved in a motor vehicle collision. He is not on a board or blocks because of dangerous conditions at the roadside with poor visibility.
What should be your first priority?

A. Tell the crew to book him into the department and you will see him when it is his turn
B. Ask the nursing staff to help you move him onto a bed
C. Immobilize the patient's neck immediately and administer oxygen
D. If the patient does not report any neck pain, ask him to move over onto the bed
E. Assess the patient's breathing and ventilation

Question 6

Which of the following statements is most accurate in describing dermatomes?

A. C6: overlies deltoid
B. T4: overlies nipple
C. T10: overlies xiphisternum
D. L4: lateral aspect of calf
E. S2: posterior thighs

Question 7

Which of the following signs has the poorest sensitivity for detecting pelvic fractures?

A. High-riding prostate
B. Perineal laceration
C. Blood at the urethral meatus
D. Blood detected on digital rectal examination
E. Instability of the bony pelvis

Question 8

Which of the following is not a definitive surgical airway?

A. Tracheostomy
B. Orotracheal tube
C. Nasotracheal tube
D. Laryngeal mask airway
E. Surgical cricothyroidotomy

Question 9

Which of the following statements is NOT true regarding the small haemothorax?

A. Bleeding is often self-limiting
B. It is usually associated with a thoracic spine fracture
C. It should be managed by inserting a large bore chest drain
D. The most common cause is laceration to an intercostal or internal mammary artery
E. Thoracotomy may be required

Question 10

Which of the following statements is TRUE regarding the assessment of the spinal cord tracts?

A. The corticospinal tract controls motor power on the contralateral side
B. The spinothalamic tract can be tested by pinprick or light touch
C. The dorsal columns consist of the fasciculus gracilis and cuneatus, and transmit crude touch afferents
D. Joint position sense is transmitted by the corticospinal tract
E. The absence of perianal sensation is known as peri-sacral sparing

Question 11

The highest achievable motor score of the Glasgow Coma Scale is:

A. 3
B. 4
C. 5
D. 6
E. 7

Question 12

Foot drop is associated with damage to which of the following nerves?

A. Common peroneal nerve
B. Femoral nerve
C. Obturator nerve
D. Posterior tibial nerve
E. Inferior gluteal nerve

Question 13

Which of the following statements regarding hypothermia is FALSE?

A. Bretylium tosylate may be effective in hypothermic arrest
B. Hypothermia is defined as a core body temperature below 35°C
C. Children are more susceptible to hypothermia than adults
D. In trauma patients, a temperature of 36.5°C should be considered hypothermic
E. Severe hypothermia is defined as a core body temperature below 30°C

Question 14

You are assessing a 49-year-old man for the need for a definitive airway.
Which of the following is not a clear indication for placement of a definitive airway?

A. Severe facial trauma
B. Risk of aspiration from bleeding or vomiting
C. Cervical spine fracture demonstrated on X-ray
D. Unconscious with a Glasgow Coma Score of 6
E. Inadequate respiratory effort

Question 15

Which of the following is typical of the chest X-ray findings associated with a pulmonary contusion?

A. Dense shadowing at the base of the affected hemithorax
B. Free air at the lung apex
C. Irregular, patchy consolidation
D. Tracheal deviation to the contralateral side
E. Widening of the mediastinum

Question 16

The following patients have sustained a head injury with a period of loss of consciousness.
In which of the following situations is immediate CT imaging not required?

A. A 60-year-old male with a fractured facial bone
B. A 65-year-old female
C. A 51-year-old male on warfarin for atrial fibrillation
D. A child that is found to have a left haemotympanum
E. A 49-year-old with two episodes of vomiting following a fall

Question 17

With regard to spine and spinal cord trauma in children, which of the following statements is FALSE?

A. Vertebral bodies are shaped like a wedge and have a propensity to slide anteriorly with flexion
B. The interspinous ligaments are more pliable than in adults
C. The zygapophyseal joints are flat
D. A child has a larger head proportionally to its body, which results in a relatively greater force on the neck with deceleration injuries
E. The conus medullaris is found at the L1–2 junction in infants

Question 18

When inserting a tube thoracostomy, one should have a sound working knowledge of the anatomy.
Which of the following statements is FALSE?

A. The neurovascular bundle runs along the inferior border, protected by the blade of the rib
B. Pectoralis major forms the anterior border of the axilla
C. The tube itself should be directed towards the diaphragmatic surface of the lung in a haemothorax
D. Insertion of the drain at the level of the nipple in males is considered safe
E. Rhomboid major forms the posterior border of the axilla

Question 19

Shooting 'electrical shock' type pains from the back to the great toe indicate compression at which anatomic level?

A. L1/2
B. S1/2
C. S3/4
D. S4/5
E. L5/S1

Question 20

Based on the following information alone, which of the following patients need not be transferred to a specialist burn centre?

A. Full thickness burn covering 5% body surface area
B. Partial thickness burns in a 48-year-old covering 9% body surface area
C. Inhalational injury
D. Significant electrical burns
E. Partial thickness burns covering the knee

Question 21

The immediate management of atlanto-occipital dislocation should involve which one of the following?

A. Spinal immobilization
B. Mayfield brace without weights
C. Mayfield brace and weights
D. Halo collar
E. Any cervical traction

Question 22

Which of the following is not a chest X-ray feature of major intrathoracic vascular injury?

A. Widened mediastinum
B. Tracheal deviation to the left
C. Oesophageal deviation to the right
D. Elevation of the right mainstem bronchus
E. Left haemothorax

Question 23

How should an oropharyngeal tube be placed in a child?

A. Insert the airway backwards, rotating the device by 180 degrees when the oropharynx is reached
B. Insert the airway on its side, rotating the device by 90 degrees when the oropharynx is reached
C. Insert the airway directly into the oropharynx
D. Do not insert an oropharyngeal airway into a child
E. There is no restriction as to how the oropharyngeal airway can be placed in a child

Question 24

Knee dislocation is characteristically associated with which of the following?

A. Superficial femoral artery damage
B. Deep peroneal nerve damage
C. Sural nerve damage
D. Chronic pain
E. All of the above

Question 25

You are about to insert an airway adjunct in a trauma patient.
Which of the following statements regarding oropharyngeal and nasopharyngeal airways is FALSE?

A. Oropharyngeal airways should not be used in the unconscious patient
B. Oropharyngeal airways in children are best inserted with the concavity facing upwards, then rotated
C. Nasopharyngeal airways should be well lubricated prior to use
D. Nasopharyngeal airways should be avoided if there is a potential basal skull fracture
E. Nasopharyngeal airways are available in different diameters and should be appropriately sized

Question 26

A 70-year-old woman is admitted with a traumatic chest injury. Her background includes chronic obstructive pulmonary disease (COPD) and ischaemic heart disease. Her initial observations are as follows: pulse 120/min, RR 25/min, BP 110/78 mmHg, oxygen saturations 83% on air.
What is your first course of action?

A. Withhold oxygen for now; she is known to have COPD
B. Give supplemental oxygen through nasal cannulae
C. Administer high-flow oxygen despite the risk of sending the patient into type II respiratory failure
D. Perform arterial blood gas analysis
E. Auscultate the lung fields

Question 27

C1 Jefferson burst fractures are characteristically caused by which one of the following mechanisms?

A. Lateral flexion
B. Forward flexion
C. Extension
D. Axial rotation
E. Axial compression

Question 28

A 67-year-old man is admitted having been thrown from a motorbike when it collided with another car. During the initial survey his airway was patent, his breathing was fast and bilateral breath sounds were heard. Chest expansion and percussion were both normal. During the primary survey his Glasgow Coma Score (GCS) falls from 13 to 8, and he is intubated. When performing a re-assessment of the patient, breath sounds are only heard from the right lung.
What is the most likely explanation for this?

A. Right-sided pneumothorax
B. Right-sided haemothorax
C. Left-sided pneumothorax
D. Left-sided haemothorax
E. Misplaced endotracheal tube

Question 29

Which of the following statements is TRUE with regard to diagnostic peritoneal lavage (DPL)?

A. Open DPL is contraindicated in patients who have had previous cardiac surgery
B. Haemorrhage as a result of the skin incision or application of local anaesthetic is unlikely to produce a falsely positive result
C. An infra-umbilical approach is preferred in advanced pregnancy
D. A retrieval volume of 20% or more of the initial 1 litre fluid volume infused into the abdomen is considered adequate
E. All of the above

Question 30

Midshaft humeral fractures are associated with damage to which nerve?

A. Axillary
B. Ulnar
C. Musculocutaneous
D. Radial
E. Median

Question 31

A lady of 31 weeks gestation is admitted following a fall. She has multiple injuries including a fractured pelvis. Her blood pressure remains low at 89/71 mmHg despite aggressive intravenous crystalloids. There are no open injuries. She begins to show signs of organ dysfunction.
What is the most appropriate initial action to take to maintain her blood pressure?

A. Begin a transfusion of packed red blood cells
B. Log roll and insert a wedge of 15 degrees with the patient in the left lateral position
C. Commence an infusion of vasopressors
D. Continue crystalloid infusion at a faster rate
E. Switch the crystalloid to a colloid infusion

Question 32

Disruption of the C1 ring can be most clearly seen on which of the following plain film views?

A. Orthopantogram (OPG)
B. Open mouth peg views
C. Lateral C-spine views
D. Skull views
E. Antero-posterior C-spine views

Question 33

You receive a trauma patient from an ambulance in the emergency department. Which of the following should you not enquire about in the emergency setting?

A. Mechanism of injury
B. Smoking history
C. Allergies
D. Past medical history
E. Drug history

Question 34

Fracture dislocations should be treated by which of the following?

A. Watching and waiting
B. Imaging then relocation
C. Relocation then imaging
D. Clinical examination and relocation, followed by imaging
E. Clinical examination and imaging, followed by relocation

Question 35

An 82-year-old man from a warden-controlled flat has fallen down a set of stairs and is accompanied by his daughter for an assessment. He has had two previous myocardial infarctions and has a below-knee amputation. The ambulance crew collected a dosette box from his house. This appears to have been infrequently used. It contains the following medications: simvastatin, furosemide and ramipril. On initial assessment you note his blood pressure to be 105/95 mmHg, pulse 95/min, oxygen saturations 96% on air and respiratory rate 22/min. Which of the following statements is not correct?

A. Blood pressure generally increases with age
B. A blood pressure of 105/95 mmHg should be considered normal in an 82-year-old
C. Pulse pressure narrows in shock
D. The patient should be reminded to take his medications today
E. Levels of serum creatinine generally stay the same with age

Question 36

Loss of respiratory function can occur with cervical spine injuries above which of the following levels?

A. C4
B. T1
C. T4
D. T6
E. T12

Question 37

Which of the following is not associated with tension pneumothorax?

A. Mechanical ventilation
B. Grossly displaced thoracic vertebrae fracture
C. Central line insertion
D. Arterial line insertion
E. Penetrating chest wall injury

Question 38

Index finger tip flexion is supplied by which of the following nerves?

A. Ulnar nerve
B. Anterior interosseous nerve
C. Radial nerve
D. Axillary nerve
E. Median nerve

Question 39

In relation to electrical burns, which of the following statements is FALSE?

A. Electrical current can be transferred through the body by ions in the extracellular fluid
B. Rhabdomyolysis should be aggressively treated with intravenous fluids
C. Mannitol is contraindicated in the treatment of rhabdomyolysis
D. Electrical burns are often more serious than the appearance of the body surface implies
E. Deep muscle necrosis can be masked by apparently normal looking overlying skin

Question 40

The transfer of a patient should be delayed until at least the prior completion of which of the following?

A. Antibiotic infusion
B. Tetanus injection
C. Secondary survey
D. Primary survey
E. Cleaning of wounds

Question 41

Atlanto-occipital dislocation should be suspected in which of the following cases?

A. To have spontaneously occurred when no other spinal injury is present
B. In shaken baby syndrome
C. With odontoid fractures
D. With C1 fractures
E. Always

Question 42

Which is the most accurate way to calculate the body surface area of burns in children?

A. Lund & Browder charts
B. Using the patient's palm (equates to 1% body surface area)
C. Wallace's 'rule of nines'
D. Measure the area with a tape measure
E. The Parkland formula

Question 43

Chance fractures are characteristically associated with which one of the following mechanisms of injury?

A. Side-on collisions
B. Head-on collisions
C. Ejection from a vehicle
D. No seatbelt being worn
E. Seatbelt injuries

Question 44

After intubation, you attempt to verify the position of the endotracheal tube. Which of the following suggests incorrect placement of an endotracheal tube?

A. Borborygmi on inspiration
B. Presence of carbon dioxide on expiration
C. Bilateral breath sounds on auscultation
D. A pCO_2 of 3.6kPa on arterial blood gas analysis
E. A midline tube noted on the chest X-ray

Question 45

Which one of the following is TRUE regarding patients with established compartment syndrome?

A. They should have continuous compartment pressure monitoring
B. They require elevation of the affected area
C. They should have hourly neuro-observations
D. They should be given morphine
E. They should undergo decompression immediately

Question 46

A 4-year-old boy is admitted to the local hospital with burns to 15% of his total body surface area. He weighs 20 kg.
How much fluid should he receive in the first 8 hours in addition to his normal maintenance demand following his injury according to the Parkland formula?

A. 300 ml
B. 450 ml
C. 600 ml
D. 750 ml
E. 900 ml

Question 47

Crush injuries can cause which of the following?

A. Metabolic alkalosis
B. Hypercalcaemia
C. Disseminated intravascular coagulation
D. Hypokalaemia
E. Respiratory acidosis

Question 48

Which of the following statements is FALSE with regard to the ageing process of the spine?

A. The water content of intervertebral discs increases with age, causing them to bulge
B. Kyphotic deformity of the spine is most marked in the thoracic spine
C. A change in the composition of the disc causes a shift of load to the facet joints and ligaments
D. Osteoarthritis is a well-recognized cause of spinal stenosis
E. The anterior longitudinal ligament is stronger than the posterior longitudinal ligament

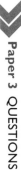

Question 49

A 2-year-old girl has knocked a kettle of boiling water onto her arm. She is admitted to the local hospital with burns covering 20% of her body surface area. She weighs 9 kg.

How much fluid should she receive in the first 8 hours following her injury in addition to her normal maintenance demand according to the Parkland formula?

A. 200 ml
B. 280 ml
C. 360 ml
D. 540 ml
E. 620 ml

Question 50

In the presence of neurological deficit, which of the following is the imaging modality of choice for further investigation?

A. MRI
B. Plain CT
C. CT myelogram
D. Plain radiographs
E. Ultrasound

6

PAPER 3 ANSWERS

Answer 1: A. The clicks of the tracheal rings are felt as the tip of the bougie passes over them

The gum elastic bougie (GEM) is a 60 cm 15 French-gauge stylette with an angled tip at the distal end. It has 10 cm graduation marks to help verify the position. Tracheal position can be confirmed by: feeling for the clicks as the angled tips rub along the cartilaginous tracheal rings; noting that the tube rotates left or right when entering a main bronchus; or noting that the tube is held up at the bronchial tree (at around 50 cm). None of these occur if the GEB is in the oesophagus. Tube position is confirmed by auscultation and capnography.

The French gauge is commonly used to describe the size of a catheter. A French gauge of *n* describes an external diameter of a $1/3n$ (in millimetres), that is, a 15 French catheter has a diameter of 5 mm. It was described by Joseph Charriere, a Parisian surgical instrument maker (1803–1876), and the unit is often therefore abbreviated to 'Ch'. So '15 French' may be written as '15 Ch'.

Bougie, from French *bougie* = candle

Answer 2: C. Vital organs are less sensitive to reduced blood flow

The ageing patient creates an additional challenge for the physician. Such patients are at an increased risk of both morbidity and mortality as a result of co-morbidities, impaired physiological reserve and the effects of ageing. In relation to the cardiovascular system, a decline in adrenoreceptors impairs the heart's ability to respond to sympathetic innervation. Throughout the body, atherosclerosis leaves vital organs at the mercy of small reductions in blood flow. The reduced ability of the lungs to oxygenate the blood compounds the tissue hypoxia already caused by impaired tissue perfusion. The kidneys are also less effective at retaining sodium and water, and are more sensitive to impaired perfusion and circulating toxins.

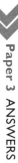

Answer 3: A. Chest drain insertion

This patient has a simple pneumothorax (there is no open wound or evidence of the pneumothorax being under tension). This results from air entering the pleural space and can occur from both penetrating and non-penetrating chest injuries (e.g. from a lung laceration). Management is by chest drain insertion without suction. Needle thoracocentesis can be considered in non-traumatic cases of simple pneumothorax. A patient with a simple pneumothorax should not be given positive pressure ventilation or be transferred via an air ambulance, until a chest drain has been inserted, due to the risk of converting a simple pneumothorax to a tension pneumothorax. Once this has been performed, air transfer is possible.

Answer 4: A. Calcification of the pineal gland

X-rays of the skull should be examined for all of the listed features. The pineal gland is only visible if calcified (which is a normal finding) and can be used to assess midline shift should it be moved away from the midline. A pepper pot skull describes multiple punched-out radiolucent lesions that usually signify multiple myeloma. The hair-on-end appearance of the skull results from prominent vertical trabeculae because of bone marrow hyperplasia. It is often associated with thalassaemia.

Answer 5: C. Immobilize the patient's neck immediately and administer oxygen

Under dangerous conditions paramedics may not be able to apply collar and blocks to immobilize a patient's C-spine. If so, this can generally be achieved within the safety of the ambulance. A more common reason for not boarding a patient would be an erroneous history. In this scenario, the patient has been involved in a significant trauma and a cervical spine injury cannot be excluded. One should immobilize the neck and apply high-flow oxygen.

Answer 6: B. T4: overlies nipple

Dermatomes are defined as areas of skin that are innervated by a specific segmental root. Clinical assessment of dermatomes can provide vital information regarding the integrity of the spinal cord. The following can be used as a guide:

- C6: thumb
- T4: overlies nipple
- T10: umbilicus
- L4: medial aspect of calf
- L5: lateral aspect of calf
- S4: perianal region

Answer 7: D. Blood detected on digital rectal examination

Although all of the listed signs should raise the suspicion of a pelvic fracture, digital rectal examination is the poorest at screening for pelvic injury. Pelvic fractures can be classified broadly into closed, open or vertical shear fractures. The latter two are associated with a poorer prognosis and, if detected, immediate steps should be taken to tamponade the bleeding by use of a pelvic binder or equivalent.

> **Shlamovitz GZ, Mower WR, Bergman J et al. Poor test characteristics for the digital rectal examination in trauma patients.** *Ann Emerg Med.* Jul 2007;50(1):25–33, 33.e1.

Answer 8: D. Laryngeal mask airway

A definitive airway is one where a tube is inserted into a trachea with an inflated cuff, with the tube subsequently attached to oxygen-enriched ventilation. Definitive airways include orotracheal and nasotracheal tubes, cricothyroidotomy and tracheostomy. The laryngeal mask airway does not pass into the trachea and hence is not a definitive airway. Although it plays a role in ventilation in trauma where definitive access is difficult, it should be upgraded to a definitive airway as soon as possible.

Answer 9: B. It is usually associated with a thoracic spine fracture

The primary cause of a small haemothorax (<1500 ml blood) is a lung laceration, or laceration of an internal mammary or intercostal vessel (penetrating or non-penetrating). It may also be associated with spinal fractures, but this is not a common association.

Bleeding is usually self-limiting and thus does not often require operative intervention, although thoracotomy may be considered if indicated. Management of acute haemothoraces that are large enough to visualize on chest X-ray is by insertion of a large bore (e.g. 36Ch) chest drain.

Answer 10: B. The spinothalamic tract can be tested by pinprick or light touch

The corticospinal tract controls motor power on the ipsilateral side. The dorsal columns transmit joint position sense (proprioception), vibration sense, and some light-touch sensation from the same side of the body. An absence of sensation is not sparing; indeed the term 'sparing' is used when a normal function is unaffected by the pathology in question.

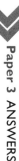

Answer 11: D. 6

The motor component of the GCS is as follows (in response to a painful stimulus):

1 No response
2 Extensor posturing
3 Flexor posturing
4 Withdrawal
5 Localizes to pain
6 Obeys commands

Answer 12: A. Common peroneal nerve

The common peroneal nerve supplies the peroneal muscles, resulting in dorsiflexion and eversion at the ankle when innervated. Damage to this nerve therefore results in a foot drop.

Answer 13: D. In trauma patients, a temperature of 36.5°C should be considered hypothermic

Hypothermia is defined as a core temperature below 35°C. It is graded as follows: mild 32°C–35°C, moderate 30°C–32°C, severe <30°C. In patients with trauma, however, a temperature below 36°C should be considered hypothermic (and below 32°C as severe hypothermia). The elderly are more susceptible to hypothermia (secondary to reduced heat production and vasoconstriction), as are children, due to a greater relative body surface area. The features of hypothermia include a reduced GCS, a grey cyanotic appearance, reduced heart rate and respiratory rate, as well as cardiac arrhythmias/asystole. Bretylium tosylate is the only dysrhythmic agent known to be effective in hypothermia but is no longer manufactured.

Answer 14: C. Cervical spine fracture demonstrated on X-ray

The indications for a definitive airway are either for airway protection or for a need to ventilate and oxygenate. Airway protection is required in the unconscious patient with severe maxillofacial injuries, where there is risk of aspiration (from blood or vomit) and with a risk of obstruction (e.g. neck haematoma, inhalation injury or laryngeal/tracheal injury). Indications for a definitive airway for ventilation and oxygenation purposes include apnoea, inadequate respiratory effort (tachypnoea, hypoxia, hypercarbia, cyanosis), severe closed head injury (when brief hyperventilation may be required) and massive blood loss. A C-spine fracture on its own is not an indication for a definitive airway.

Answer 15: C. Irregular, patchy consolidation

Pulmonary contusions are the most common potentially lethal chest injury and may be associated with a flail chest. A respiratory failure develops over time and patients should be monitored closely. The presence of significant hypoxia (pO_2 <8.6kPa or SaO_2 <90%) may require intubation and ventilation. Chest X-ray typically shows air-space consolidation that is irregular and patchy, or homogenous and diffuse.

Answer 16: A. A 60-year-old male with a fractured facial bone

Fractures of the facial bones alone (not to be confused with skull fractures) are not an indication for immediate CT imaging. However, a thorough evaluation of the patient should be sought to assess for other clinical features that might. It is worthy to note that all patients who are 65 years of age or above presenting with a head injury with associated loss of consciousness require CT imaging according to the National Institute for Health and Clinical Excellence (NICE) guidelines.

Answer 17: E. The conus medullaris is found at the L1–2 junction in infants

The conus medullaris (conical tip of the spinal cord before becoming the cauda equina) ends at the L1–2 junction in adults. In children, it is proportionally longer. As the skeleton grows at a faster rate than the spinal cord, the cord appears to finish more cephalad as the child grows into adulthood. The conus medullaris would be expected to lie at L2 or L3 in an infant.

Answer 18: E. Rhomboid major forms the posterior border of the axilla

Chest drains should be inserted into the affected hemithorax within the safe triangle. The anterior border of the axilla, the mid-axillary line and the sixth rib bound this triangle. The insertion site should be just above the superior border of the rib to avoid neurovascular damage. A chest radiograph should always be taken to confirm the tube's position after the procedure. It is lattisimus dorsi that forms the posterior border of the axilla, not rhomboid major.

Answer 19: E. L5/S1

These symptoms are characteristic of L5/S1 nerve root compression.

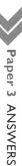

Answer 20: B. Partial thickness burns in a 48-year-old covering 9% body surface area

Transfer to a specialist burn unit can improve patient outcomes. All of the above, with the exception of option B, should be transferred if possible. Typically, a patient less than 50 years of age with partial thickness burns less than 20% need not be transferred providing there is no other reason for doing so.

Answer 21: A. Spinal immobilization

Traction following atlanto-occipital dislocation is contraindicated. Spinal immobilization is indicated initially. Subsequent relocation may be performed under anaesthetic by spinal surgeons.

Answer 22: B. Tracheal deviation to the left

Tracheal deviation to the right is an X-ray feature following major vascular injury in the chest. A widened mediastinum is the most reliable feature. Other chest X-ray features include: obliteration of the aortic knob, oesophageal deviation to the right, depression of the left mainstem bronchus, elevation of the right mainstem bronchus, left haemothorax and fractures of the first or second rib.

Answer 23: C. Insert the airway directly into the oropharynx

Oropharyngeal tubes should only be inserted in an unconscious child. They should be sized appropriately and inserted in the same orientation in which they will eventually sit. This is to reduce the risk of tearing friable soft tissues within the oropharynx that can lead to further airway compromise. Remember, a tongue blade might prove useful.

Answer 24: D. Chronic pain

The high-energy injury resulting in complete dislocation of the knee carries a very high morbidity and is associated with significant injuries to surrounding structures, including the popliteal artery, common peroneal nerve and cruciate and collateral ligaments. Patients are at significant risk of developing chronic pain from such an injury.

Answer 25: B. Oropharyngeal airways in children are best inserted with the concavity facing upwards, then rotated

Oropharyngeal airways must not be used in conscious patients, due to the risk of gagging with subsequent vomiting and aspiration. Oropharyngeal airways can either be inserted with the concavity facing downwards, or with the concavity facing upwards until the soft palate is reached, before rotating it 180 degrees. However, the latter method should be avoided in children as rotation of the device can cause damage to the mouth and pharynx.

Nasopharyngeal airways are inserted into one nostril and should be appropriately lubricated and sized (e.g. the same diameter as the patient's little finger). These airways should be avoided in patients with a potential basal skull fracture, as there is a risk that the tube will pass directly through the cribriform plate and into the skull vault.

Answer 26: C. Administer high-flow oxygen despite the risk of sending the patient into type II respiratory failure

This question is testing an appreciation of CO_2 retainers. A minority of COPD patients are chronic retainers of CO_2 and rely on a level of oxygen insufficiency to stimulate breathing.

Ventilation is controlled by central and peripheral chemoreceptors in the floor of the fourth ventricle and the carotid bodies respectively. Owing to CSF lacking protein and haemoglobin, changes in pH (and CO_2) are poorly buffered. Small fluctuations in pH are therefore rapidly detected, which sparks an alteration in ventilation and normalization of pH. Chronic elevation in CO_2 desensitizes this central feedback. The resultant dependence of peripheral chemoreceptors means that ventilation is initiated by hypoxia and not CO_2. In such patients, administering supplemental oxygen can impede respiratory drive and induce a respiratory acidosis and respiratory failure.

However, in an emergency situation, high-flow oxygen should be given. Patients in the acute setting die from hypoxia, not from hypercarbia. Retention of CO_2 can be corrected by either invasive or non-invasive ventilation at a later stage.

If the patient deteriorates and is in imminent respiratory failure, they should be intubated and ventilated mechanically.

Answer 27: E. Axial compression

Extreme axial loading results in the C1 ring being disrupted. This can occur following a large weight being dropped on the head or the patient landing directly on the head following a fall.

Answer 28: E. Misplaced endotracheal tube

It is not uncommon for the right main bronchus to be intubated instead of the trachea. This occurs on the right more frequently than the left because there is a sharper angle made between the left bronchus and the trachea. Correct positioning of the endotracheal tube should be confirmed before concluding the patient has developed a new pathology.

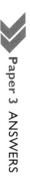

Answer 29: D. A retrieval volume of 20% or more of the initial 1 litre fluid volume infused into the abdomen is considered adequate

Open DPL is contraindicated in patients with previous abdominal surgery as the presence of adhesions can reduce the validity of the test. Haemorrhage during the incision is a real concern and in patients with pelvic fractures and advanced pregnancy; a supra (not infra) umbilical approach is recommended to avoid damage to a gravid uterus or entering a large pelvic haematoma.

Answer 30: D. Radial

The radial nerve spirals around the midshaft of the humerus prior to piercing the intermuscular septum before entering the forearm. It is vulnerable to fractures of the humeral shaft.

Answer 31: B. Log roll and insert a wedge of 15 degrees with the patient in the left lateral position

Heavily gravid women should be placed in a tilted position to the left lateral side to relieve the pressure exerted on the inferior vena cava from the uterus. This is a fast and effective method of improving venous return and therefore cardiac output (Starling's law). Vasopressors should be a last resort as their adrenoceptor action restricts blood flow to the uterus and will starve the foetus of oxygen. Continued infusions of crystalloid or colloids for that matter can lead to dilutional anaemia. Therefore, if tilting the patient to 15 degrees and administering a second fluid challenge has been ineffectual, a transfusion of packed red blood cells should be administered.

Answer 32: B. Open mouth peg views

Fractures of the C1 ring can be best seen on C1/C2 open mouth views. This reveals displacement of the lateral masses. Further imaging using CT is required to better define the fracture.

Answer 33: E. Drug history

An AMPLE history should be obtained: allergies, medications, past medical history, last time of eating and drinking, exposure and mechanisms of injury.

Answer 34: D. Clinical examination and relocation, followed by imaging

Fracture dislocations are associated with significant neurovascular compromise. Urgent relocation should be the priority following evaluation. In the presence of neurovascular compromise, there should be no delay while imaging is sought.

Answer 35: A. Blood pressure generally increases with age

Careful consideration should be made in the interpretation of blood pressure in elderly patients, many of whom have systemic hypertension (as implied by the ramipril in this scenario). Such a patient may normally maintain a blood pressure far exceeding that considered normal and a reading of 105/95 mmHg may represent a significant fall in circulating volume. Be rigorous in your assessment of blood loss and consider the early use of supplemental tools such as a FAST scan for excluding occult bleeding.

Answer 36: A. C4

Provided there is innervation of the diaphragm, ventilation should continue despite loss of thoracic innervation for rib expansion. The innervation for the diaphragm arises from the C3, C4 and C5 nerve roots, so an injury above the C5 level can compromise respiration. Remember, C3, 4, 5 keeps the diaphragm alive.

Answer 37: D. Arterial line insertion

All of the given options, with the exception of arterial line insertion, are associated with tension pneumothoraces. Arterial lines are generally sited well away from the thorax, such as at the arm or forearm. The most common cause of tensioning is positive pressure ventilation when used in the management of visceral pleural injury. A tension pneumothorax impedes venous return by compression of the vena cava. By Starling's law, this reduces cardiac output and can lead to imminent death.

Answer 38: B. Anterior interosseous nerve

The anterior interosseous nerve supplies index finger tip flexion as well as supplying flexors to the thumb, index and long fingers and pronator quadratus.

Answer 39: C. Mannitol is contraindicated in the treatment of rhabdomyolysis

Rhabdomyolysis is a condition characterized by the destruction of skeletal muscle. The myoglobin that is released from muscle is nephrotoxic and can induce acute renal failure. It should be managed with aggressive fluid resuscitation and careful fluid balance. The diuretic mannitol can be used in the treatment of rhabdomyolysis and drive a diuresis.

Answer 40: D. Primary survey

The primary survey must be carried out before transfer. The completion of the secondary survey, wound cleaning, antibiotics and tetanus prophylaxis can be delayed in cases where urgent transfer is required.

Answer 41: B. In shaken baby syndrome

Atlanto-occipital dislocation is usually incompatible with life unless resuscitation is available immediately at the scene. It has been shown to be present with around 19% of fatal cervical injuries. It is to be suspected with shaken baby syndrome when the victim dies immediately after shaking.

Answer 42: A. Lund & Browder charts

Lund & Browder charts are widely used in clinical practice and offer an accurate way of assessing the percentage body surface area of burns. Areas of skin with erythema and no blistering should not be included in the calculation. Wallace's 'rule of nines' is easier to remember and use, but less accurate. Knowing that the surface area of the patient's palm equates to 1% of the total body surface area can also be useful.

Once the percentage body surface area of burn is known, an accurate calculation can be made of the volume of fluid that should be used for resuscitation. The Parkland formula can be used for this.

Answer 43: E. Seatbelt injuries

Chance fractures are transverse fractures through the vertebral body and are characteristically caused by seatbelt injuries. They are associated with retroperitoneal and abdominal visceral injuries.

Answer 44: A. Borborygmi on inspiration

Following insertion of the orotracheal tube, the cuff is inflated and ventilation commenced. Capnography, or a colorimetric CO_2 monitoring device, helps confirm correct positioning by detecting the presence of CO_2 in exhaled air. Further evidence for correct positioning can be gained from chest auscultation (bilateral equal breath sounds) and chest X-ray findings. A raised pCO_2 may suggest inadequate ventilation, but the pCO_2 of 3.6 kPa is normal. The presence of borborygmi in the epigastrium on inspiration suggests oesophageal intubation.

Borborygmi, from Greek *borborygmos*, is an onomatopoetically coined word for intestinal rumblings.

Answer 45: E. They should undergo decompression immediately

Established compartment syndrome is a surgical emergency requiring urgent fasciotomies to release the compartment pressure. There must be no delay. This is a limb-threatening injury.

Answer 46: C. 600 ml

The Parkland formula is given by:

Volume of Ringer's lactate over 24 hours = Percentage burn × Weight (kg) × 4 ml

In this case:

Percentage burn × Weight (kg) × 4 ml = 15% × 20 kg × 4 ml = 1200 ml over 24 hours

Half of the total volume of fluid should be given over the first 8 hours. The second half of the fluid should be given over the 16 hours.

½ × 1200 ml = 600 ml (over first 8 hours)

Note: This volume of fluid will be in addition to the patient's normal maintenance demands.

The Parkland formula was devised in 1968 by the American physician Charles Rufus Baxter (1930–2005), working at the Parkland Memorial Hospital in Dallas.

Answer 47: C. Disseminated intravascular coagulation

Rhabdomyolysis can cause hypovolaemia, metabolic acidosis (with a compensatory respiratory alkalosis), hyperkalaemia and hypocalcaemia, as well as disseminated intravascular coagulation.

Answer 48: A. The water content of intervertebral discs increases with age, causing them to bulge

The ageing process of the vertebral column renders the elderly patient vulnerable to injury and consequently spinal cord damage. With age the intervertebral disc loses proteoglycans and water. This makes the disc less pliable and the annulus fibrosis more susceptible to rupture. Herniation of the disc predominantly occurs

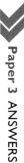
posterolaterally. This is because the anterior longitudinal ligament is broader and more fibrous than that of the posterior longitudinal ligament.

Answer 49: C. 360 ml

The Parkland formula is given by:

Volume of Ringer's lactate over 24 hours = Percentage burn × Weight (kg) × 4 ml

In this case:

Percentage burns × Weight (kg) × 4 ml = 20% × 9 kg × 4 ml = 720 ml over 24 hours

Half of the total volume of fluid should be given over the first 8 hours. The second half of the fluid should be given over the 16 hours.

$$\frac{1}{2} \times 720 \text{ ml} = 360 \text{ ml (over first 8 hours)}$$

Note: This volume of fluid will be in addition to the patient's normal maintenance demands.

Answer 50: A. MRI

In the trauma setting, MRI is indicated to ascertain the extent of compressive lesions such as haematoma, herniated disc, contusions and/or disruption of the spinal cord.